T0192748

Consumerism in the Human Services

David P. Moxley

Consumerism in the Human Services

Rationale, Evolution, Perspectives, and Policy Strategies

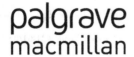

David P. Moxley
University of Alaska Anchorage
Anchorage, AK, USA

ISBN 978-981-16-7194-4   ISBN 978-981-16-7192-0   (eBook)
https://doi.org/10.1007/978-981-16-7192-0

This Palgrave Macmillan imprint is published by the registered company Springer Nature Singapore Pte Ltd.
The registered company address is: 152 Beach Road, #21-01/04 Gateway East, Singapore 189721, Singapore

To my students, past and present, who have sharpened my thinking by asking "what do you mean?" I affirm you all.

Abstract

In this Palgrave Pilot, I offer a typology capturing the diversification of contemporary human service systems based on four system cultures, each framing a distinctive way of understanding how consumers and survivors influence systems of care. The typology, formed through two principal dimensions, involving the extent to which consumers or survivors control the outcomes and processes of support, captures the scope of contemporary human services, whether those are within mental health, aging, immigration, corrections, health, developmental disabilities, assistance to veterans, or child welfare.

For each of the four types, involving professional dominance, enabling, recipient-centered, and person-controlled cultures, I consider how each variant reveals the principal qualities consumers and survivors introduce into human service systems. Employing the four types as heuristic frameworks, I offer specific strategies for how values and innovations that stand as alternatives to traditional professional dominance can shape human service systems. I conclude the monograph with a consideration of the future of consumerism.

Throughout the monograph, I underscore the significance of consumerist strategies in human services. By making consumer roles explicit, and/or by amplifying voice and dissent within human services, those who create, implement, and develop those systems can come to offer a range of options for the people they wish to assist without necessarily assuming total control inherent in professional dominance or neglecting people by abandoning them to their own devices too often with few or no resources.

Too often what social work and other helping disciplines or professions assert as evidence-based is a product of professional control over systems and practices. Consumers, and survivors, can introduce considerable innovation into systems, oftentimes making professionals late adopters of practices those consumers initiate and use in action. Ultimately in this monograph, I seek to offer a framework of consumerism that speaks to diverse ways of providing support to people imbuing consumerism with multiple cultures, and multiple expressions. Such a framework implicates a number of ways of shaping contemporary social welfare and human management policies, ones I offer as policy choices.

Contents

List of Figures

1

Rationale for Consumerism in the Human Services

Introduction

At least since the 1960s, consumerism has been an integral part of society, the development of which parallels the great social movements in the early and latter part of the twentieth century. Consumerism, encompassing ideas like adequate information about products people use for various reasons, some life sustaining like pharmaceuticals, or essential to mobility, like automobiles, emerges from the early twentieth century, particularly when the so-called Muckraker journalists, labor activists, and activist scientists and social scientists questioned the authority of the private sector to produce how they wished as well as the governmental officials who had a responsibility for protecting people from the dangers inherent in poorly conceived or manufactured products (Nader, 2012).

Consumerism raises the bar considerably in shaping if not specifying the relationship between people and governments. One of the milestones in the history of consumerism in society took place when Ralph Nader took the national stage in the United States condemning the Corvair automobile in his book, *Unsafe at Any Speed*. Nader's work ignited the consumer movement in the United States that would then catalyze

© The Author(s), under exclusive license to Springer Nature Singapore Pte Ltd. 2021 1
D. P. Moxley, *Consumerism in the Human Services*,
https://doi.org/10.1007/978-981-16-7192-0_1

consumerism broadly and consumer movements in specific areas of society, as well, including voting rights, medicine, mental health or psychiatric care, aging, developmental disabilities, and education. Nader's work brought into public awareness what would emerge as a novel idea, but one steeped in the values of American constitutionalism: that consumers had rights, and those rights extended to the protection of their safety and well-being. Nader's work built on an early movement in the United States involving regulation of corporations (Roosevelt, 2012).

Some would say Nader single handedly created consumerism as a new social institution within American society and even internationally, at least in the so-called developed world in which affluence produced a plethora of products through innovations in manufacturing, and even in other areas of modern living, such as health care. He also created a new profession of sorts found in public interest activism. Empowerment of consumer role can be seen in Nader's seminal advocacy: he defined within society the modern conception of active consumers who have rights to be both informed about the products and services they consume and protected against dangerous business practices (Nader et al., 1976). The activist role of Nader probably is underappreciated. His work anticipated the mushrooming of various protest movements and of self-help and mutual aid activities emerging during the 1960s, which stretched well into the 1970s. In this sense, consumerism was not tied to an activist government, but expanded to include public systems, like higher education, and nonprofit or nongovernmental organizations.

For perhaps the first time in history, university faculties of law and their students, journalists, professionals from diverse backgrounds, and nonprofit organizations became interested collectively and collaboratively in the rights of ordinary consumers. The protection of consumers through public interest advocacy became well established and professionals from myriad disciplines aligned with public interest lawyers to ferret out the violations of established consumer rights and foster the expansion of such rights. Advocacy within the disability fields is linked with human rights to produce empowerment options for people who were likely unwanted within a society prioritizing good looks, acceptable bodies, and expensive accoutrements.

The activism of later consumer advocates reflects Nader's inspiration. Elizabeth Warren's efforts to create the Consumer Financial Protection Bureau captured the spirit of consumer protection, especially of groups whose members could be victimized by unscrupulous business practices in credit card, payday loans, and retail or health domains. Her work, emerging during the Great Recession of 2008, found a sympathetic ally in the Obama Administration, but would soon be vitiated by a subsequent presidential administration that sought to weaken consumer protections. Still, her predecessor in the United States Senate, Barney Frank, pursued reform of banking and financial policies to benefit consumers (Weisberg, 2009).

Recent movements within public health and food safety also reflect Nader's influences, particularly in the area of consumer protection. Risk communication about food security have resulted in numerous recalls of foodstuffs, and a movement to label processed food reflects societal efforts to support informed consumer choice and health promotion. Still, movement to apply the same labeling that accompanies foodstuffs to pharmaceuticals is a low-key effort that can inform consumers considerably. A movement to promote health literacy also is occurring. All of these movements seek the empowerment of consumers using enhanced labeling, information, and methods for supporting the interpretation of information that is sensitive to the reading and information processing skills of diverse consumers.

A Naderistic conception of consumer role suggests an active, discerning, and assertive consumer who could and should question what was being received and how one was being treated. Nader legitimized an assertive consumer in all sectors of society. And, the conception of consumer role offered people an opportunity to define their own expectations about products and services, ones too often provided in unregulated markets, or closed systems in which business professionals and their marketing allies came to dominate decision-making (Nader, 1967).

Public Interest Law and Rights Protection

The ethos and knowledge base of public interest law also influenced human services stimulating innovation in rights and altering profoundly the relationships between human service or medical professionals and the voluntary or involuntary recipients who received care from them. Prior to legislation in the United States, case law began to alter the sanctity of professionals, particularly in areas like mental retardation and psychiatric disability. An activist judiciary was on the cutting edge of a consumerism to protect people with disabilities, particularly those who were under the care (or control) of state institutions (Yarbrough, 1981). The indictment of care undertaken by journalists in particular resulting in exposes produced either in book-length treatments of institutional abuse, newspaper accounts, or in other media forms brought professional hegemony, abuse, and neglect into the minds of the general public.

Exposes like Willowbrook State School undertaken by activist social scientists like Burton Blatt, and journalists like Geraldo Rivera, revealed the intimate details of the neglect of children with mental retardation who were under state care. Legislators, particularly congressional ones in the United States, could not overlook their responsibilities for addressing such neglect and abuse for the very institutions, journalists, social scientists, and lawyers were exposing received federal funding. Bobby Kennedy, in particular, took interest in the Willowbrook scandal given the location of the institution within the state of New York, which he represented in the United States Senate.

Those exposes, ones indicting the adequacy of social care arrangements for people with disabilities, particularly severe ones, that placed them under the authority of state government in the United States, further catalyzed consumerism, a form of public activism in the United States that invented rights protection and advocacy systems for a range of populations like people living with developmental disabilities and other cognitive limitations, physical disabilities, psychiatric impairment, and aging. The rights protection and advocacy movement in the United States came to offer a principal rationale for consumerism in human services: that professionals were not unbridled decision-makers who could act without accountability. Related here was yet another rationale: the entirety of professional knowledge itself was limited, and professionals, especially medical ones, could not act with impunity ignoring the very rights of people whose treatment or care they managed.

Echoing here were ideas of Nuremberg in which Nazi physicians were placed on trial for the misuse of professional knowledge. The Nuremberg provisions, which would come to profoundly influence the treatment of participants in both medical and social research in the United States, further empowered the status of the consumer as a participant in federally funded research. The idea of informed consent would come to alter the relationships between researchers and those who participated in the research, which is now well established in law and regulation in the United States.

The emergence of rights protection and advocacy as a visible product of consumerism in the United States also stimulated other protections human service consumers could trigger to process either concerns, complaints, or violations, particularly within the context of social or health services in which they possess a vested interest and therefore should expect substantive due process.

Structures like ombudsmen offices, rights officers, compliance officers, and internal rights protection capacities within public bureaucracies responsible for the delivery of social services serve as reminders and examples that people in need can trigger their dissatisfaction with public services and their treatment within public bureaucracies. Indeed, visible on the walls of those facilities operated by bureaucracies should be explicit statements of consumer or client rights, and recipients should receive paperwork and brochures listing those rights and how to process concerns, register their dissatisfaction, or make formal complaints. Those rights may include incorporating factors pertaining to race, religion, veteran status, physical characteristics, sexual orientation, marital status, or gender identity.

The expansion of these qualities that create protected populations (i.e., protected by law as classes) over time means that consumerism has been both increasingly inclusive and specific in their prioritization of particular groups. Social institutions and their bureaucratic expressions are powerful in determining the quality of life of people, and in degrading people's lives (Douglas, 1986). This inclusivity offers yet another rationale for consumerism in the human services: that institutions providing human services should be neither arbitrary nor discriminatory in responding to people whose qualities are immaterial to the supports, services, or opportunities those institutions offer. Consumerism strives to limit discrimination. It recognizes if not institutionalizes diversity as an essential condition to which public institutions must be responsive.

Factors Promoting Recipient Use and Control over Human Services

Still other values come into play when considering institutional responsiveness. Accessibility of care or services, transparency of performance information, alternative options of care, and opportunities for people to refuse certain forms of care become important values operating within the scope of consumerism. And, responsiveness can come into play through the actual diversity policies of a given organization when its administrators, leaders, and service providers are mindful of the importance of matching the social attachments of providers with those of recipients. Race, gender identity, sexual orientation, and cultural identity, manifest in overt clothing or rituals or bodily features of those offering social services, may serve as important ways of further realizing accessibility. Responsiveness may demand that human service organizations connect with the people they seek to engage and assist in ways reflecting a greater cultural strategy within communities or societies.

Ultimately, responsiveness may be more voluntary than legalistic. It can involve the suitability of architecture, furnishings, art and decoration, use of time, celebrations, and overt monuments to build a strong and positive relationship with those who form the recipient population that human service organizations seek to assist. Here consumerism can extend to building faith people invest in the organization, trust between recipients and helpers, and community assets in which people take pride in the organization as an essential utility or asset within the community. The idea that the organization is "ours and for our community" may be an essential sentiment in which recipients expect and experience respect and dignity when they transact care with a given organization. Respect and dignity may stand as the most important values of consumerism, particularly for those people or groups who experience considerable marginalization and oppression in their daily lives (Kateb, 2011; Rosen, 2012; Waldron, 2015).

Empowering the Status of Recipients and Consumers

Formalistic elements of consumerism will likely amplify the rights governing the relationships of recipients to public bureaucracies or organizations receiving public funding. Those formalistic elements implicate the recipients' awareness of their rights, policies guaranteeing those rights, procedures for affirming those rights in action, or potential or real violations of rights, and processes for advancing those rights. These elements operate in rights protection and advocacy as a cornerstone structure of human services, especially in the public sector inclusive of organizations that receive public funding or possess a publicly legislated charter. These formalistic elements are essential as the basis of consumer empowerment since without them recipients have little recourse for advancing their dissatisfaction.

Interest in how recipients experience the organization reflected in their satisfaction imbues them with a level of standing within that organization. Without this standing, recipients are likely involved in cultures of helping that reduce their status. Cultures that marginalize the status of recipients, or that frame that status using pejorative stereotypes, are likely system-centric. In this characterization, the system exists for itself, diminishes the status of its users, and engages in rituals that essentially control or better manage the people who look to it for benefits. This is a critical stance on my part. But such system behavior is indicative of street-level bureaucracies that are too often overwhelmed by the severity of issues recipients bring. In system-centric cultures, consumerism is likely highly proceduralized, and the leadership of such organizations may discourage the voice of recipients about their treatment or care.

Consumerism and Organizational Culture

Alternatively, human service organizations that invest considerably in amplifying the voice of recipients offer a culture that one could character-ize as either consumer-centric or consumer-driven. Those cultures foster voice on the part of the people they serve, and would likely strengthen formalistic elements of consumerism that government or accreditation may stipulate and heighten ones the organization undertakes on a volun-tary basis.

Voluntary elements are part of an organization's intentional engage-ment in building consumer culture oftentimes manifest as community building among those who hold status as providers (who may actually be former or current recipients in some cases) and those who stand as recipi-ents of care, treatment, or support. As I emphasize above, the voluntary elements can be comprehensive and pervade the organization as a whole system of care and support. This comprehensiveness is part of a design in which the two values of respect and dignity orchestrate internal beliefs, attitudes, values, and artifacts, what Schein (2016) calls organizational culture, into a positive framework of collaboration among those who are in helping roles and those who are in recipient roles.

The rationale for consumerism is steeped in organizational culture, given that most societies organize helping resources as formal entities in the public, private, or nongovernmental spheres. So, consumer culture can matter given the importance many societies place on providing social and health services through formal organizational structures. This ratio-nale recognizes the importance of recipient status, which can be dimin-ished by society, valorized within group life, or diminished by organizations. Forces diminishing the status of recipients are widespread in most societies. Individuals in need may experience diminished status because gatekeepers, people in authority, those in direct contact with such individuals, and/or members of the general public see them as unworthy, dangerous, child-like, or impure. Public judgment of impurity may factor into the creation of diminished status in critical ways, producing stigma, the spoiling of identities, and the seclusion of people who are different. Many social movements move against rigid conceptions of purity that limit the freedom and well-being of their members (Shotwell, 2016). However, social institutions can channel public bias reinforcing ideas about social risk—who is to be feared? And, who is to be accepted or emulated? (Douglas, 1982).

People in need of formal assistance may be seen as "the other" who cannot fulfill societal expectations for autonomy, independence, and self-sufficiency, which of course can implicate stigma. Majority perceptions of rules and their violation may set in motion forces, particularly moral attitudes, ones that result in diminished status of those who do not have access to basic resources. The societal assignment of the cause of human problems to those who experience the consequences of those problems is highly prevalent in many social welfare cultures. Indeed, societal members may interpret consequences that people bear as the causes of the problems individuals with diminished status experience. Such an inequity reflects "blaming the victim" (Ryan, 1976).

Countering Cultural Preferences and Finding Alternatives to Normative Aesthetics

Ultimately, one of the most serious violations involves impurity when a person is seen as dangerous because their body or psyche is infected, the infection can pass to others, and the person lacks a mindfulness to control their conduct or behavior, thereby making them behaviorally unpredictable. A societal judgment of impurity can further marginalize someone and result in their isolation as a result of an enforced or informal exile from human groups. Perhaps the most serious consequence of a societal determination of impurity is enforced separation from mainstream society that occurs through incarceration, geographic segregation, or extreme deprivation resulting in serious impairment or even death.

Consumerism in this context expresses itself as a means of status elevation. At least people who experience diminished status in the general society can experience empowered statuses and roles within the very organizations designed to help them. In this way, organizational culture matters, and it matters a lot. System-centric organizations prize the operation of the system over the status of the people to whom they offer help. Consumer-centric organizations may come to appreciate how their cultures not only valorize consumer roles, but also use the culture itself to protect people from external social forces bringing about insult and outright abuse. A person who is struggling with an infectious disease likely can benefit from support, hospitality, and a valorization of their efforts to maintain their health. They do not need an additional burden from a society that condemns them for being ill. Consumerism can come to incorporate such protection, strengthened through the orchestration of symbols of defiance (Jones, 2000).

Aesthetics introduce the idea of beauty and the sublime. The bucolic community of support nested in the mountains of a forested region can serve restorative purposes for people who have known only deprivation if not cruelty. There are such intentional communities around the world the purpose of which is to restore human well-being through person-to-person interactions with nature and wildlife. Those communities introduce the sublime through their architecture and their juxtaposition with the natural world. The aesthetic can be integral to the restorative process because it nurtures sensory experience in the most positive way, and fosters sensuality, which itself can calm those whose prior degradation emanates from considerable and complex trauma.

The mainstream values informing aesthetics, however, may not fit all people, since their bodies or physical forms, sensory experiences, and relationship to society may be unfavorable for them. For the layperson, such people may be expendable, marginal, or even useless. They may not have the qualities that the general society favors and, therefore, they experience rejection or are simply ignored. The members of such groups can introduce their own aesthetic useful in organizing for them that which is cool, beautiful, or wonderful. Let me refer to this as the counter-aesthetic since it counters what the mainstream considers as the principal organizing aesthetic of society.

We witness a normative aesthetic in advertisements, commercial products, and norms and rituals that enforce acceptable ways of being in society. It comes in the form of proper hairstyles, proper hair quality, cosmetics, clothing, housing, and street addresses or zip codes. The counter-aesthetic moves against such normative prescriptions. It can open up other ways of being and becoming as those who experience marginalization form their own norms, and interactional rules. They form their own contexts favoring the ways they wish to function, and they may eschew mainstream institutions, like the work ethic, in favor of other avenues of productivity.

Intentional communities may embody a counter-aesthetic in which their members or residents create their own organizations, communities, neighborhoods, and support systems. My prediction is that given a narrow and confining aesthetic operative in the general society, people who "do not fit" such a prevailing notion of beauty will create their own options and opportunities. Following the dicta of Marcus Aurelius, the great Roman Emperor who was an adherent to Stoicism, in which he said "It is up to you," those who form a counter-aesthetic produce forms of self-help and mutual support that address their needs perhaps independent of the general society. Disability activists who may invoke the South African disability rights motto "Nothing about us, without us," may further speak to an organizing construct one could come to appreciate as a counter-aesthetic (Charlton, 2000). "Do not impose either your will or your values on us." Such libertarian ideology speaks to the idea of unfettered freedom: we will do things our way.

One can also think of the negative aesthetic. Here the prevailing aesthetic is inaccessible to those who experience harsh treatment by the general society and its agents, such as human service, law enforcement, or justice officials. The negative or brute aesthetic imbues places and people with degradation, threat, or danger. Cells in degraded architectures like prisons or other systems of incarceration, or degraded housing, can capture the negative aesthetic (Pitzer, 2017). Previously, I suggest that positive aesthetics, that which bring beauty and the sublime into people's lives, are essential to positive human development. Degraded human development is the product of the brute, so visible in Brute Art in which one can witness tortured souls, the distortion of the body, the destruction of mind and sensory perception, and the degradation of nature and animals (Eco, 2007).

One may come to think of the brute as an individual matter. The person is ugly, and this is a personal attribute or quality, perhaps reflective of deeper moral or ethical flaws, or a product of misfortune. Brute art, however, underscores the reality of institutionalized ugliness. But my interpretation is that such art is not making statements about individuals. It is making statements about people in situations, contexts, or circumstances. It is society's mistreatment that instills ugliness. And, ugliness here forms the negative aesthetic—one that harms people or dispossesses them of what is essential to the flourishing of human beings: a form of aesthetic that prizes a social death.

Some commentators may speak to how negative or brute aesthetics can call forth the best in human spirit. They point to the heroic—the person who resists, who transcends, and who emerges from the degradation more whole or even better than when they entered the mess from which the negative aesthetic forms. For me, the heroic serves societal aims of institutionalized neglect.

What does the aesthetic have to do with consumerism in human services? Aesthetics is inextricably linked with human development in a very positive sense, or with its degradation in a very negative sense. The exposure to a positive aesthetic, especially one formed through the interactions of people, animals, architecture, private and public spaces, and nature, can empower the human spirit and raise life-affirming and life-enhancing questions about possibilities and horizons for those who compose such an aesthetic and those who experience it. The anti-aesthetic can spur human creativity in the face of opposing social forces. Novel or original forms of human and community support and interactions can follow from such creative action. Brute or negative aesthetic impoverishes or destroys human development and its possibilities even though a lone hero may transcend such a mess.

The heroic is fine, and is important enough across cultures to serve as a principal form in the humanities. Yet, civilization can ask for more. Consistent with a human rights framework, we understand the consequences of trauma, deprivation, torture, and abandonment (Felice, 1996; Rieff, 2002). With such knowledge, people can demand more, and ask for better. They can demand a base level of decency, and a life without oppression. They can expect that dignity and decency can create for them a positive outlook manifest in the now of optimism and hope for the near and distal future. Ultimately, such expectations are fundamental to consumerism—people can expect more out of life, and a better existence, if not now, then for the future. If not for themselves, then for their loved ones and compatriots.

Differentiating Voice and Dissent

I can broaden the rationale for consumerism in the human services when we take into consideration two forms of action on part of those who are marginalized. Those involve what Hirschman (1970) calls voice and dissent. In the previous discussion I invoke a rationale for consumerism steeped in voice. Mechanisms whether societal or organizational amplify the voice of the recipients who can use formal rights mechanisms or those voluntary ones an organization incorporates to elevate the status of the consumer. Likely designed to maintain recipients in social or health service systems, the amplification of recipient voice can result in considerable alteration of human services, the augmentation of supports, development of new opportunities, and an alteration in the roles of those who are recipients.

Politically those kinds of changes focus on reform and for policy making such changes seek more responsiveness to recipients. In this manner, organizations can become more consumer-centric or even consumer-driven in terms of the control recipients can exercise over the means of assistance they receive. Such reform can ensure the stability of existing organizations as recipients become active consumers in the affairs of human service systems. Some organizational cultures may narrow those opportunities of involvement by focusing them on a particular kind of activity or role, such as an expansion of recipient participation in hiring decisions. Some organizational cultures may expand those opportunities considerably adding role elements that stretch from governance to direct delivery of care to other recipients. Nonetheless, the expansion of recipient roles may be a central reform policy governing many human service systems.

Dissent, however, takes consumerism in a different direction. Through this mechanism, people who otherwise could be seen as recipients leave human service organizations intentionally because they see those very organizations as the source of the problems they experience. Dissent comes about when the response to the social issues people experience are factors defining the problematic circumstances people experience. Withdrawal from the role of recipient, a break in ties with particular human service organizations, a disavowal of the legitimacy of reform, and a dismissal of the relevance of human service professionals may be part of a larger radical strategy of social activism among those who do not see such formal means of helping as legitimate.

Those advancing dissent may work to influence the reallocation of human service funding to dissenters themselves, the creation of alternative support systems outside of human service systems, and the prevention of governmental or societal intrusion into the lives of people manifest when the greater society seeks to enforce some form of unwanted or unacceptable human management. Indeed, for dissenters, human services are about human management in which the greater society seeks to bring certain groups under intentional control.

Neglect, abuse, or dismissal may influence or otherwise bring about dissent on the part of people who grow intolerant of established human service entities and the policies enfranchising their work and operations. Instructive here is the history of mental retardation in the United States and the treatment of children and their parents who had no claims on educational systems for appropriate support of children with disabilities. Prior to the authorization of Public Law 94-142, the Education of All Handicapped Children's Act, parents would likely experience rejection by local school systems whose representatives would not accept children because of their mental retardation arguing that they could not benefit from primary school education, or that the schools themselves lacked the capacities to educate children with cognitive limitations.

This rejection occurred in the face of the realities that parents paid local taxes in support of public education and their children were denied what came to be known as a "free and appropriate public education." Those parents founded their own schools, oftentimes in the basements of churches, and served as their children's educators portending charter schools or even homeschooling that exists today. Charter schools and homeschooling reflect forms of dissent in which families that do not wish to be involved in public schools withdraw into alternative structures. Movements to found academies focusing on addressing the needs of children with minority status, like Hispanic or African American children, reflect the kind of dissent inherent in an active culture of consumerism within society. That mainstream institutions fail to meet the needs of particular groups, offers a strong rationale for a form of consumerism based on dissent.

Some human service entities may dismiss certain groups of recipients because of behavioral, conduct, or other kinds of qualities those organizations find unacceptable. Those individuals may collectively resist such rejection and agitate for acceptance by those organizations oftentimes using legal mechanisms to gain a hearing and achieve their ends. But some groups may simply withdraw and exercise dissent through the founding of alternative support systems. These individuals may consider themselves survivors of the existing system, and the alternative support system may incorporate a narrative that separates them ideologically from existing human service arrangements within the community.

Such an alternative narrative may be highly visible in the support systems founded by ex-patients of mental health systems, those who found intolerable the actions of those systems in abridging their rights, well-being, or freedom. One can argue that undergirding dissent is the value of self-determination. Particularly in democracies that prize market mechanisms as a means of responding to consumer needs, people should control those resources otherwise mediated through formal human service organizations to address their needs, and create support systems that work for them. Using vouchers or purchase of service arrangements can foster such self-determination introducing market mechanisms into human service systems. Vouchers, however, may not cover the full costs of social support people require, and may be inadequate in addressing the social integration costs people or families may require to ensure true participation in a given institution, like schools, rehabilitation services, or employment opportunities.

Two Vectors of Consumerism

The distinction between voice and dissent can create two different vectors of consumerism in the human services (and in social welfare at a policy level and human services at program levels). The amplification of recipient voice within human service organizations can produce a reform strategy restructuring organizations internally through the alteration of relationships between providers and recipients, and through the diversification of support arrangements internally as organizations seek to be more responsive to the daily living needs or aspirations of recipients. A mental health organization may add employment services and supports, housing options, and educational options as a result of its personnel becoming increasingly responsive to the people the organization assists.

The organization may adopt a recovery model as a way of supporting people living with severe and persistent mental health issues and, as a result, alter the ideology and culture of service delivery. As a result, based on the interests and wishes of the people it assists, the mental health organization may reduce its investment in rehabilitation processes. Alternatively, it may increase its investment in helping people address the alteration they are experiencing in their identities and sense of self as they gain control over their illnesses and grapple with challenges inherent in autonomy and independence.

This kind of consumerism favors informed, active, and assertive recipients who form collaborative relationships with the professionals who assist them, and who are involved in making social support occur in the lives of the recipient population of the organization. Bolstered by a strong rights framework within the organization, but supported by an equally strong or even stronger voluntary culture of responsiveness, this form of consumerism seeks to empower and elevate the status of people whose previous status was degraded if not diminished. For these recipients, consumerism means choice, participation, involvement, and perhaps even control over their primary organizational experience as recipients. Empowerment within such a culture emerges from an elevated status in which organizational culture expands the role set available to recipients, and valorizes the status of those receiving assistance.

Those involved in expressing and acting on dissent operate within a framework of consumerism. But this form of consumerism is more consistent with economic conceptions. Those who engage in dissent remove themselves from one set of transactions and markets to engage in an alternative form of transaction within quasi-markets. Here, rather than using the idea of role expansion, perhaps a more accurate conception is role innovation. Sociologically, these actors are more like social innovators or even social entrepreneurs who are creating new forms of social relationships outside of established and acceptable modes.

As a result, novel or innovative forms of action may emerge, ones less reliant or even nonreliant on the prevailing paradigm operating in human services in which professionals may be more dominant than recipients. Those who dissent may come to see themselves as survivors of the existing system who are out on their own to create new support systems. As survivors they live in ways they find satisfying, or they engage in careers critiquing the systems from which they have withdrawn, or agitating for a change in existing arrangements within human services. Rather than be informed, active and assertive like consumers, dissidents as survivors may introduce the very ideas needed to create considerable innovation. Indeed, dissenters as survivors may prefigure arrangements in the present that human service systems may embrace in the future. Human service professionals may be late adopters arriving at arrangements survivors conceived of and enacted in a previous generation.

Conclusion

In closing, the reform strategies of consumers can leave in place the existing organizational structures characteristic of contemporary human service systems. I refer to these strategies as *progressive*. Alternatively, a consumerism of dissent offers *radical* implications because they remove actors from existing systems and hold the potential for changing substantively the relationship between society and citizens, particularly those whom the greater society may consider unwanted.

In a grander political view, a consumerism of collectivism involves individuals heightening their claims for support in the greater society.

They may want safer, more, or better in the supports that the society offers them. These provisions can come in the form of regulations empowering the status of human service consumers, and valorizing their identities. Becoming a citizen or having the provisions of citizenship, such as in the cases of refugees, trafficking victims, or immigrants, means, for me, that dignity is the basis of consumerism in the human services. As Rosen (2012) explains, central to dignity is the human desire to make claims.

Alternatively, consumerism in a libertarian stance likely calls forth a freedom from society's unreasonable regulations and restrictions. "Leave me to my own devices, leave me alone, and do not abuse my rights." Here inherent rights, may be natural ones, coalesce to protect the person's integrity, perhaps best achieved through integration of rights and identity, and expand a person's scope of agency within a society. "Do not restrict me because of what you see as something you do not like or want in the society." Here is a different dignity than one emanating from collectivism. It is a dignity grounded in personhood, and in personal agency and responsibility for self and one's actions.

References

Charlton, J. (2000). *Nothing about us without us: Disability oppression and empowerment*. University of California Press.

Douglas, M. (1982). *Risk and culture*. University of California Press.

Douglas, M. (1986). *How institutions think*. Syracuse University Press.

Eco, U. (2007). *On ugliness*. Rizzoli.

Felice, W. (1996). *Taking suffering seriously: The importance of collective human rights*. SUNY Press.

Hirschman, A. O. (1970). *Exit, voice, and loyalty: Responses to decline in firms, organizations and states*. Harvard University Press.

Jones, C. (2000). *The making of an activist: Stitching a revolution*. Harper.

Kateb, G. (2011). *Human dignity*. Belknap Harvard.

Nader, R. (1967). Keynote address presented to the consumer assembly. In R. Nader (Ed.), *The ralph Nader reader*. Seven Stories Press.

Nader, R. (2012). Unsafe at any speed. In E. Bruun & J. Crosby (Eds.), *The American experience: The history and culture of the United States*. Black Dog & Leventhal Press.

Nader, R., Green, M., & Seligman, J. (1976). Who rules the giant corporation? *Business and Society Review*, Summer.

Pitzer, A. (2017). *One long night: A global history of concentration campus*. Little, Brown.

Rieff, D. (2002). *A bed for the night: Humanitarianism in crisis*. Simon & Schuster.

Roosevelt, T. (2012). The national should assume power of regulation over all corporations. In E. Bruun & J. Crosby (Eds.), *The American experience: The history and culture of the United States*. Black Dog & Leventhal Press.

Rosen, M. (2012). *Dignity: Its history and meaning*. Harvard University Press.

Ryan, W. (1976). *Blaming the victim* (Revised and updated edition). Vintage.

Schein, E. (with Peter Schein) (2016). *Organizational leadership and culture* (5th ed.). Wiley.

Shotwell, A. (2016). *Against purity: Living ethically in compromised times*. University of Minnesota Press.

Waldron, J. (2015). *Dignity, rank, and rights*. New York.

Weisberg, S. E. (2009). *Barney Frank*. University of Massachusetts Press.

Yarbrough, T. (1981). *Judge Frank Johnson and human rights in Alabama*. University of Alabama Press.

2

Evolution of Consumerism in the Human Services

Introduction

Those who are unfamiliar with consumerism in the human services may find its rich and encompassing qualities as a surprise. Those who are familiar will find in this chapter some justification for viewing consumerism as an essential feature within and outside of human service systems. Consumerism has established self-help and mutual support as fundamental building blocks of such systems, and it augments the assertiveness of those who change their roles in relationship to professionals. Consumerism introduces those who otherwise would be subordinate to professionals to new kinds of statuses and roles. Consumers themselves may serve as providers within human services, and survivors can take adversarial positions against prevailing policies, and challenge the ways human services can manage people and abrogate their freedom.

Indeed, consumers or survivors may emerge as serious policy advocates, and family members of patients or clients may engage in their own form of advocacy with primary interests in serving as front-line caregivers. Advocacy undertaken by family members may clash with advocacy undertaken by consumers, survivors, or professionals. All four interest

© The Author(s), under exclusive license to Springer Nature Singapore Pte Ltd. 2021
D. P. Moxley, *Consumerism in the Human Services*,
https://doi.org/10.1007/978-981-16-7192-0_2

groups may create temporary coalitions working together to bring about forms of social change their members agree upon. Those coalitions may be somewhat fragile, disappearing when the various groups achieve their interests, and then recrystallizing when opportunities for policy advocacy remerge.

Contemporary human service systems are likely amalgams of diverse interests—those reflecting the preferences of consumers, survivors, family members, or professionals, who themselves may be diverse based on life experiences, perspectives, knowledge, identities, functions, and role legitimization. This evolution is the result of considerable activism and policy innovation during the latter part of the twentieth century. The consumerism of the twenty-first century has benefited from this evolution. Human services now incorporate at least six functionalities indicative of the diversity of consumerism:

1. The withdrawal of people from human services, to found their own support systems outside of the boundaries of officially sanctioned systems, and/or to establish a critical posture against what the members perceive as professional intrusion into their personal lives.
2. A conscious and purposeful expansion of consumers' roles beyond that of patient or client to incorporate helping, support, and assistance roles, some well-established within human service systems, or some merely amounting to token forms.
3. An empowerment of consumer roles within zones systems would traditionally reserve for leaders within the community that do not identify as consumers or survivors. These roles can include consumer involvement in organizational processes, system oversight and monitoring, policymaking commissions, evaluation, and accreditation.
4. The legitimization of credentials that are not necessarily a product of education and specialized training to encompass experiences consumers have had within systems that facilitate the formation of specialized knowledge in relationship to that system. Experiences as a recipient of HIV case management, for example, can imbue that person with considerable knowledge about effective and ineffective practice.
5. The transactional aspects of self-help and mutual support that can produce benefits for everyone involved in those transactions in the

production of support, psychological security, and informational competence.

6. The augmentation of rights that foster access to what recipients want for themselves, and to foster refusal of assistance professionals may assert as necessary or good.

Some Significant Historical Roots

Innovation in consumerism is not a new concept. There are traces of advocacy in social policy and human service innovation and reform as far back as the eighteenth century when Pinel, a French physician, introduced humane treatment and care of people confined to psychiatric institutions. Pinel was an innovator in what came to be known as moral treatment involving the support of people with psychiatric illness to engage in the regularities of daily life with support and kindness offered by caretakers, typically the staff of institutions.

In the United States, Dorthea Dix came to advocate for the advancement of psychiatric care by bringing it under the umbrella of the federal government, a noble effort but one that failed. Pinel's and Dix's efforts as well as those of other advocates sought to humanize care of people who had originally been objects of ridicule and physical abuse, and institutional abuse within the British Poor House system, the remnants of which the United States embraced in its institutional models, particularly facilities for people with mental retardation.

Working in tandem with Adolf Meyer, the advocate of a public mental hygiene movement, Clifford Beers, himself a former psychiatric patient, worked to advance human service systems during the early part of the twentieth century (Dain, 1980). I refer to mental hygiene as human services since the movement itself sought to build relationships between community-based clinics and schools, between those clinics and court systems, and between clinics and health providers. Meyer's idea of mental health was expansionary and addressed multiple forms of prevention anticipating the public health movement in mental health that would come together under the leadership of First Lady Roslyn Carter in the United States, and manifest itself in the Mental Health Systems Act of

1980. Carter sought to harmonize mental and public health systems within regional authorities. Her leadership anticipated the long-running search for parity among mental health and physical health financing, something that continues to challenge policymakers to this day.

The efforts of Beers resulted in the formation of state and local mental health associations, which amplified the voices of primary consumers, family members as secondary consumers, and enlightened professionals. Beers sought to improve care within state institutions, and did not focus on mutual support and self-help as augmentations of systems of care, or as primary responses in and of themselves. Beers's efforts as an advocate intersected with those of Meyer further reinforcing the primacy of professional intervention. In the context of professional intervention, within mental hygiene, a model of multidisciplinary practice emerges legitimizing the involvement of multiple professions each contributing something distinctive to formal treatment of people coping with various issues of daily life, many emanating from the stresses and deprivations of poverty.

Beers could not influence dramatically the reform of state institutions, which continued to offer merely custodial care (since the ideas of active treatment and the developmental model were far in the future), and he could not prevent abuse and neglect within such institutions. It is Beers, however, that stood as an exemplar of consumer activism. A former patient himself, Beers was sensitive to how society treated people with serious health issues, particularly those who could not speak on their own behalf (Beers, 1907). He worked in collaboration with professionals, engaging in efforts to expand public awareness of mistreatment.

Consumerism expanded as the twentieth century progressed. Again, in the domain of serious mental illness, the emergence of social clubs came about through innovations in institutional care, and then subsequently in community contexts. Models like the WANA Society (We Are Not Alone), a consumer movement emerging from the early throes of institutional reform mid-century, and jump starting the clubhouse movement and its variations. In the United States, *Action for Mental Health*, a report published in 1961 by the federal Joint Commission on Mental Illness and Health, recognized the contributions of ex-patient groups to primary care and community support. The report identified four kinds of ex-patient alternatives inclusive of social clubs, Mental Health Aid Societies, therapy groups, like Recovery, Inc., and social rehabilitation centers.

The authors of *Action for Mental Health* failed to see consumers as autonomous of professionals. They were to serve in adjunct roles and operate in subordinate ways to medical and rehabilitation professionals. Although *Action for Mental Health* called attention to the importance of these structures and their members in the provision of mental health and human services, they were not primary. Professionals served in primary roles, and consumers were relegated to subordinate ones.

The model of the club operated in other domains among people who were blind, or deafened or hard of hearing. Largely those clubs emerge within the state school systems for the blind and deaf fostering close ties among students within those schools, and fostering ties in the form of social support, romantic attachments, and business formation among graduates. These clubs incorporate self-determination and empowerment values since they make the members central to the functioning of a club, and members controlled their programs and built their cultures.

Such associations anticipate a much broader membership movement in human services, in which people would come to eschew the status of patient or even client, and would come to define their own agency as central to helping themselves and their fellow members. The membership model incorporates group work as its own movement within human services. Theorists and practitioners of group work underscore the healing and recovery powers of group life and assign to cohesion and interpersonal support considerable influence as agents in helping people cope with issues they face. The membership model would come to build on the core qualities of group work and then bring it into the development of milieus, communities of support, and intentional communities.

Clubs as a predecessor to a more expansionary consumer movement are significant for several reasons. First, they offered forms of support that professionals failed to consider or felt were outside of their roles as formally educated professionals. Second, they were under the control of their membership who could decide how they would offer support to members. Third, they filled gaps in human service systems in which people would otherwise become isolated. Indeed, consumerism in the human services holds a significant role in filling such gaps, particularly those forming when people sought support during long stretches of time when they were without professional assistance. In filling those gaps, consumers often engaged in innovation in formulating ways of helping one another.

In spite of the domain in which clubs operate, they underscore the importance of social support for people who experience stigma and related marginalization, and isolation. It is very interesting that clubs as paradigm emerge when the literature on social support expands, especially through the work of Gerald Caplan (1974). His basic and applied research on social support recognized the importance of diverse support in fostering human well-being, and enduring theme of the social sciences and the helping professions. Caplan was one of the first researchers to offer a general theory of social support, one identifying the importance of stress buffering for people who are experiencing considerable social change manifest in alteration of their roles such as during divorce, grief, social displacement like unemployment, and economic change. Caplan also anticipated the powerful influence of social support on primary and secondary prevention in the helping professions (Caplan, 1964).

Social support is a critical concept within consumerism since it recognizes that through stigma, discrimination, and prejudice, whole groups can experience marginalization, and an accompanying deprivation. Recognition of the beneficial aspects of the peer group emerge during World War II, the Korean Conflict, and the 1950s and 1960s in the United States and internationally. The knowledge of the importance of self-help to recover from short- or long-term combat situations underscored the important role of the peer group as a provider of social support. Social support became instrumental in supportive group interventions to resolve crises, and address so-called battle fatigue, the forerunner diagnosis to PTSD. Self-help and mutual support became important tools in the provision of care at front-line hospitals, particularly within Mobile Army Surgical Hospitals, or what were called MASH units in the Korean conflict, a model that remains useful in the treatment of combat exposed military personnel engaged in contemporary conflicts.

The influence of social support would take on more significance as a tool for helping people in the resolution or mitigation of crisis, and negotiate successfully role change, institutional change, and social change. Inspired by Caplan's work, researchers would come to further differentiate social support into multiple types like emotional, instrumental, and informational, and into mediation through psychological factors, and social network factors. The broad scope of social support, its dynamics, and its consequences is now a mainstay of social and behavioral inquiry, particularly in understanding the mediating influences of what social researchers call strong and weak ties within social networks.

Moving across the divide of mid-century, in the late 1960s, social policy recognizes the influence of diversity and indigenous perspectives on the provision of human services. Legitimization of paraprofessional roles, outreach workers, and what Brager (1965) called the indigenous workers came to change human service systems, but only peripherally. Such policies changed the personnel qualities of human services, in which the introduction of indigenous workers reflected those qualities, typically demographic, of the communities in which the systems operated. Power, however, remained with formally educated and credentialed professionals, and it was their hegemony that would soon foster an ex-patient or survivor movement. What Brager came to call indigenous nonprofessionals served as ways of making human service systems more responsive to the users of human services, and also produced an alternative pathway for members of local communities in which systems operated to make them more reflective demographically of users. These roles anticipated the current peer support movement in recovery.

The Ex-Patient Movement and the Two Vectors of Consumerism

The idea of the ex-patient of the 1950s, which meant the person who completed a regimen of psychiatric treatment, took a profound shift in the 1960s and 1970s, as individuals grossly dissatisfied, even horrified, by their treatment within psychiatric institutions, began to organize alternative support systems, reflective of a movement in which activists expressed their dissent at the unrestricted dominance of psychiatrists, and mental health professionals (Chamberlin, 1978). Within the general protest movements dominating the 1960s, and early 1970s, the ex-patient movement took root. The movement fostered support systems that could serve as alternatives to established community mental health programs, and psychiatric treatment.

Alternatives like drop-in centers, crash pads, drug-free support systems, and consciousness-raising support groups emerged across North America. Infused with an anti-psychiatry ideology that was informed by ideologies created by innovators in other protest movements, like feminism, civil rights, disability rights, and Gay rights, the anti-psychiatry movement challenged existing dominance of medical professionals. Unlike the original clubhouse model and peer support options that the Joint Commission identified, those involved in ex-patient alternatives viewed themselves as part of a larger struggle for human and social rights. These organizations and their participants vehemently upheld their ideologies even in the face of tremendous delegitimization within American psychiatry.

The requirement within psychiatry that patients be passive, the ex-patient movement sought to empower its members, and support their assertiveness. Protest, withdrawal, critique, and innovation in support were the practices characteristic of the movement. Those qualities themselves could be observed in other movements, especially Black empowerment, and Feminism. The movement's literature, one of criticism and critique, came to frame existing human services as not only problematic but also oppressive and evil.

The indictment of these systems was supported by civil rights attorneys and programs, including the emergence in the United States of the Protection and Advocacy for Mentally Ill Act signed into law by George HW Bush, who also supported the passage of the Americans with Disabilities Act. That these pieces of legislation coincided expressed the tension of the day. Following on the heels of tremendous activism by disability rights advocates, those two policies reinforced both libertarian and collectivist ideals. People deserved fair and appropriate treatment, and they were free to refuse treatment.

Libertarian views frequently operate within consumerism. The best regulation is minimal regulation, according to those advocates for maximum liberty and freedom within a given society. Government intrusion into the lives of people is an evil, and citizens should be wary of such a form of social control. From a collectivist perspective, however, people should not be without the support they seek for themselves. Collectivism suggests access to what Gil (1998) came to call life-sustaining resources and what twenty-first-century social theorists would come to call those social systems that bring people above the threshold of deprivation and poverty. That libertarian ideas would synergize with collectivist ones is paradoxically reflective of the robust framework of consumerism in the human services.

In the history of social rights in mental health and psychiatric treatment, the label of ex-patient possessed double meaning: a situation that reflects the duality of consumerism. It literally means supporting people who are former patients of institutional care to live in community settings. Shaping the image of the patient are biomedical constructs involving ill health, dependency, and disability. Alternatively, the label of ex-patient suggests an individual who stands in opposition to contemporary human service arrangements and ideologies. Social constructs shape the image of the person, as well as their social identities, involving first-hand experience of discrimination, prejudice, stigma, social intolerance, and repressive social norms.

Placing the second use of ex-patient into socio-legal and political contexts, society creates a dual challenge. First, if they underscore the idea of vulnerability of people with various disabilities as limiting their potential, then the society itself becomes responsible for enhancing social and community support. This means that those individuals should have access to the necessities of daily life without bureaucratic entanglements they too often experience.

Such care involves both individualized and normative considerations. On the one hand, someone deserves forms of care governed by individual considerations, which was itself a product of litigation by rights advocates in the early 1970s. On the other hand, people deserve social provisions available to all citizens. Weaknesses in either response mitigates the quality of support people should experience given the label that society imposes. In this sense, equity involves a societal recognition that labeling comes with considerable negative consequences and, as a result, can prevent people from achieving what in contemporary social development calls inclusion. Inclusion means that people can enjoy the fruits of societal participation in what everyone should have: a right to work, housing, recreation, education, and good health care. Within the United States, inclusion and normalization link into a potential social policy system that speaks to opportunities people can access to advance their autonomy, independence, and dignity.

Second, people who are so labeled should command a range of rights that prevent the overreaching by a society that fears people who are different. A label can damage both individual standing and reputation. It can abridge social mobility and personal autonomy. From a libertarian stance, such consequences implicate the erosion of civil rights.

Consumerism within the mental health and psychiatric domains form a tension between social provision and the rights governing quality of care, quality of life, and civil rights, those consistent with the Bill of Rights of the United States Constitution. Consumerism reflects a Jeffersonian ideal in which people have standing in a society and they should enjoy a modicum of prosperity. That consumerism possesses two vectors reflects the complexity of this concept within human service systems.

Consumerism in Corrections and Substance Use Treatment

One can appreciate how the duality of the ex-patient movement operates in other sectors of human services. Corrections in the early part of the twentieth century witnessed efforts by reform-oriented penologists and wardens to engage in institutional reform through the expansion of the roles of inmates. As warden of Sing Sing prison in 1914, Thomas Mott Osborne introduced the idea of self-government through what was called the Mutual Welfare League. Although this innovation was short-lived since Osborne's tenure was cut short, his efforts sought to expand the typical role prisons assigned to inmates by offering them opportunities to participate in the operation of a facility.

Later in the century, a 1969 federal court decision eliminated a prison regulation that prevented the involvement of prisoners in helping one another. If this regulation had prevailed, prisoners would have been prevented from accessing essential legal services through self-help and mutual aid. It would have prevented prisoners from using "jailhouse" legal skills to assist their peers. The jailhouse lawyer stands as an exemplar of how those who hold a diminished status can gain the knowledge and competencies typically reserved for professionals and exercise these in potentially effective ways. It also reflects the important role people can play in assisting their peers through mutual aid, especially when professionals are unavailable or unwilling or unmotivated to lend assistance.

Allen's seminal book, published in 1981, addresses the shift in consumerism within corrections. He documents the decline of rehabilitation and a shift to punishment. Gone was the idea of active assistance within corrections settings even though remnants remain. The emergence of drug use as a criminal offense in the United States reinforced punishment. Paradoxically, whole communities were drained of adults, particularly in African American communities as American penal policy shifted to offer re-entry programs within those communities after they were decimated by the penal policy. The "war on drugs" became the war on Black women and men, with a child welfare system responding to incarceration through the provision of social services to Black children.

The substance abuse treatment domain faces a duality of focus implicating both criminalization of users and the provision of therapeutic and recovery assistance. Substance use treatment now has a long history of using peer support to facilitate recovery and relapse prevention. Peers are actively involved in harm reduction efforts, and peers serve important roles in the rehabilitation continuum. A key credential for many substance use treatment systems is experience in the use of substances, treatment success, and active maintenance of recovery. Those credentials recognize success in overcoming addiction, which suggests a social learning component of recovery. Peers learn from those helpers who have primary experience and who know first-hand the process of personal recovery and its many challenges and setbacks. Such personal experience can be an element of certification programs.

Consumerism here reflects an aim to reduce the social distance that can separate the recipient from the helper. Mutual identification between the recipient and helper (i.e., the recipient sees the helper as someone who understands the "ropes," and the helper understands the real-life obstacles that the recipient must negotiate) may actually be a defining characteristic of consumer role innovation. A bureaucracy can easily compromise this central characteristic when professionals fail to see consumers as a significant reference group (Lipsky, 1980).

This idea of linking consumerism with humanization of human service systems emerges ostensibly as a social innovation in the 1960s. Previously I mention Brager's notion of the indigenous worker in human services, a role also proposed by Pearl and Riesman (1965). With the aim of making social services more accessible and responsive to people in poverty, these scholars invoked three challenges that social services faced: (1) professionals were not likely of the communities in which they worked, (2) the number of trained human service professionals were limited in any given system, and (3) considerable social distance likely existed between trained professionals and the people they sought to assist.

The considerable social distance meant that professionals were limited in their capacities to be sensitive to social class, ethnic, racial, and language differences between helpers and recipients. Pearl and Riessman and Brager proposed the "indigenous nonprofessional" or the "helper therapist," as useful roles in offering more psychological access to a system, and immediate responses by those individuals who a community would more likely trust than a human service professional who community members saw as different or even alien.

Theoretically, the indigenous worker could serve as an advocate to address those needs professionals may overlook since the latter may want to protect their own interests, career and organizational ones. Professionals themselves could overlook the needs of a given community since as contrasted with the indigenous worker, they likely did not identify with that community, or even reside within it (Levinson & Schiller, 1966).

As I indicate in substance use treatment, and with the theoretical models of the 1960s, the intent here is to foster a strong identification between the recipient and the worker. According to Pearl and Riessman, the incumbent of such roles could model recovery, increase motivation of consumers to seek treatment, and communicate more effectively with recipients than professionals, thereby improving recipients' psychological comfort with workers, and fostering trust. These kinds of arrangements were visible in a number of 1960s models of social services in the United States emerging during the "War on Poverty" of the 1960s. These included Welfare Rights Organizations whose members served as advocates for welfare recipients within social service bureaucracies (Mayer, 1972), Mobilization for Youth (Fishman et al., 1965), child welfare (Costin, 1967), aging social services (Farrar & Hemmy, 1963), and community action agencies (Gordon, 1965).

Members of the movement here were seeking ways of responding to diversity and to the overrepresentation of people of color living in poverty who were populating the rolls of community service organizations. Throughout the United States in the 1960s, and into the early 1970s, public interest attorneys were fighting court battles in which they sought to define the receipt of human and social services as a property right. But if those individuals found such assistance to be inaccessible, then organizational cultures vitiated the right through lack of access and the absence of relevance. Innovation in consumerism in this period involved the creation of new kinds of helping roles reserved for people with the "right kind" of social attachments (especially in terms of class, race, and ethnicity) as a principal strategy of mitigating inaccessibility.

A consistency here across all sectors of human services is that the systems themselves define innovation as creation of new roles based on a social theory of action the aim of which is to humanize the system itself. For these movements, a principal tactic is to alter the characteristics of those who provide assistance directly to people in need. Ultimately, as a consequence of such efforts, people would find the system more accessible, sensitive to their needs, and responsive to their social attachments, such as racial, ethnic, sexual, or class identities. As the social movements of the 1960s and early 1970s lost their luster, such efforts began to wane even though some systems retain such roles, such as in contemporary mental health organizations.

Larger Scale Social Movements

Three consumer innovations here are worth noting in terms of their incorporation of the paradigm of an assertive consumer. ADAPT, a grass-roots organization founded in the United States, engages in disability rights promotion and is directed against those organizations or institutions that limit people's access to essential life opportunities. ADAPT incorporates both self-help and mutual support for group members who also engage in civil disobedience collectively to overcome societal discrimination and oppression. Members risk arrest for their efforts to make visible the injustices people with disabilities face in their daily lives. ADAPT illustrates how a voluntary group of activists can use civil disobedience in shaping local disability policy.

A second innovation is the emergence of support systems operated for and by people with physical disabilities. Here the independent living movement is worthy of note. The prototype of this programmatic form is seen in the Berkeley Independent Living Center. Originating on the campus of the University of California at Berkeley, it emerged out of a protest movement led by people with physical disabilities (Shapiro, 1993). Consumers diffused this model to address access, mobility, housing, and social and employment barriers facing members of the disability community.

The concept of an independent living center run by and for members was grounded in self-help and mutual aid, two factors frequently emerging within the consumer movement in human services. That this model operated independently of human service professionals reveals the duality of independence. First, members undertake efforts to support themselves on their own, a form of independence from a dependence on a system of care, and second, the center supports independence as a valued societal aim many if not all people hold in common.

ACT-UP reflects a third social innovation worth noting, which involved activism advancing sexual orientation and its intersection with health policy. Gay activists engaged in civil disobedience, policy advocacy, and agitation to alter dramatically National Institutes of Health policy toward clinical trials for AIDS medication. That the National

Institutes of Health altered its clinical trial protocol, brought the voice of people with AIDS and their advocates into the upper reaches of health policy, and supported the testing of alternative medication or treatments. The founding of ACT-UP in 1987 reflected social activism on part of people coping with AIDS and its vastly negative consequences.

The organization emerged from the Lesbian and Gay Community Services Center. Located in downtown Manhattan, New York City, the center offered sanctuary and protection from the negative reaction by the greater society toward Lesbian and Gay people and reflects the powerful influence of the membership model on efforts to produce collective well-being for and by a group whose status society can dramatically and substantially compromise. As a membership organization, the center could advance Gay and Lesbian culture, develop social services responsive to people's culture and identities, and support socialization and social support among members.

Movements in domestic violence, sexual assault, and sex education have been important influences in shaping consumerism. Early work among those who have experienced domestic violence and sexual assault resulted in multiple innovative models facilitating safety and protection among those experiencing violence, and in the recovery process itself. The peer movement in sex education has equipped teens as peer support specialists bringing important information about disease prevention, safe sex, pregnancy prevention, consent, and awareness to groups whose members would not respond readily to adult professionals.

The women's movement has been instrumental in framing the importance of mutual support and consciousness raising in liberating a specific group from institutional dominance in which sexism is one of the most virulent dynamics. Feminism has come to redefine and reframe many movements and their methodologies including the empowerment of roles, dramatic alteration in roles, the development of alternative support systems, and the creation of opportunity structures, all based on an encompassing critique of male dominance within society. Today societies across the globe are witnessing the emergence of new norms governing interactions between groups within communities, the world of work, and the operation of households. And, movements like Me Too and Black Lives Matter reflect assertive consumerism within society: they reinforce how society's neglect of multiple groups can result in considerable psychological, social, and economic harm for whole classes of people. Such neglect can also result in death.

Conclusion

From the standpoint of mutual assistance within consumerism, societal dynamics and the evolution of societies are likely shaping a more empowered consumer in multiple areas of group life. Such assistance can foster the development of cultures that move against the greater ills of a society, and that protect members, advance their identities, and provide well-needed social support in the face of marginalization, abuse, rejection, and oppression.

Group life can raise consciousness of members about what constitutes a "personal problem" perhaps helping members understand that their actual problems are situated in the greater society, ones perpetuated by social structures, poorly performing institutions, and the abridgment of rights. Groups and the organizations they can found as innovative alternative structures within a society can make clear the dynamics of sexism, racism, handicapism, or other social dynamics that threaten well-being on personal and group levels. That these problems are not the making of the members is a vital product of consciousness raising fostering the actions these members undertake to support one another, and perhaps change society itself. Group life becomes a critical bulwark against oppression.

This chapter does capture how consumerism cuts across society, and makes visible the dysfunctional conduct of societal institutions and their representatives as a principal reason supporting the existence of consumerism. The history of consumerism reveals its evolution within multiple domains. Fueled by social movements, key actors, and social innovation, consumerism is situated in status and role change that particular groups advance in their quest to find equity or equality in reluctant societies. They may search for such equity within human service systems that may be willing to offer new roles for consumers. Or those groups may simply not recognize human service systems as the venues for supporting their identities. In such cases, they may seek support among members and operate outside of human service systems exercising withdrawal as an expression of dissent.

References

Allen, F. (1981). *The decline of the rehabilitative ideal: Penal policy and social purpose*. New Haven: Yale University Press.

Beers, C. (1907). *A mind that found itself*. New York, NY: Doubleday.

Brager, G. (1965). The indigenous worker: A new approach for the social work technician. Social Work, 33–40.

Caplan, G. (1964). *Principles of preventive psychiatry*. Basic Books.

Caplan, G. (1974). *Support systems and community mental health*. Behavioral Publications.

Chamberlin, J. (1978). On our own: patient-controlled alternatives to the mental health system. New York, NY: McGraw-Hill.

Costin, L. (1967). Training nonrprofessionals for child welfare service. *Children, 13*(2), 63–68.

Dain, N. (1980). *Clifford W. Beers: Advocate for the Insane*. University of Pittsburgh Press.

Farrar, M., & Hemmy, M. (1963). Use of nonprofessional staff in work with the aged, Social Work, 44–50.

Fishman, J. R., Pearl, A., & MacLennan, B. (1965). New careers: Ways out of poverty for disadvantaged youth. Report of conference sponosored by Howard University Center for Youth and Community Studies. Washington DC.

Gil, D. (1998). Confronting injustice and oppression. New York, NY: Columbia University Press.

Gordon, J. (1965). Project Cause: The federal antipoverty program and some implications of subprofessional training, *American Psychologist, 20*(5).

Lipsky, M. (1980). Street-level bureaucracy: Dilemmas of the individual in public services. New York, NY: Russell Sage Foundation.

Levinson, P., & Schiller, J. (1966). Role analysis of the indigenous nonprofessional. *Social Work, 2*(3), 1–10.

Mayer, R. R. (1972). Social planning and social change. Englewood Cliffs, NJ: Prentice-Hall.

Pearl, A., & Reissman, F. (1965). New careers for the poor. New York, NY: Free Press.

Shapiro, J. P. (1993). No pity: People with disabilities forging a new civil rights movement. New York, NY: Times Books.

3

Substantive Differences Between Consumerism and Survivorship

Introduction

The typology I offer in the subsequent section, composed of two dimensions, and four corresponding quadrants, captures how I have come to organize or otherwise conceive of the various cultures composing contemporary human service systems. The existence of innovations in care both within and outside of human service systems is a testimony to the considerable diversification of those systems or evidence that those systems could not offer the kinds of support people needed or sought for themselves exclusively through professional assistance (Mowbray et al., 1997). Consumers and survivors have sought to establish ways of offering support but directed to contrasting ends and likely fueled by contrasting conceptions of need and status than what human service system can offer solely through professionals.

© The Author(s), under exclusive license to Springer Nature Singapore Pte Ltd. 2021
D. P. Moxley, *Consumerism in the Human Services*,
https://doi.org/10.1007/978-981-16-7192-0_3

Consumerism and Role Expansion

Consumerism is itself a legitimization of established human service systems that structure the relationship between providers and recipients in hierarchical forms. There are likely at least three aspects to this structure: (1) empowerment of the role, decision scope, and substantive decisions over which people in human service systems could exercise control, (2) role expansion in which recipients in human services could engage in the provision of support to others, particularly the provision of peer support, self-help, and mutual support, and (3) leadership roles in which people in human services could hold influential positions involving governance, policymaking, program planning, and evaluation (Mowbray et al., 2001).

Consumerism is linked to social role expansion by the established system offering recipients opportunities to assist their peers. In American society people who are marginalized and face oppressive societal forces can experience diminished status. Status is diminished when some people especially those with particular qualities fall out of the mainstream, because of limited resources and marginalization. Within American society, illness and poor health can limit the adequacy of resources, those generated particularly through workforce participation, and resource limitations can compromise social integration or full inclusion. Limited social integration can aggravate stigma and deviance, which in turn can further limit social integration creating a vicious cycle. The presence of stigma and deviance, and those factors compounding it, are largely secondary considerations within human service systems. Illness, impairment, and disability—their diagnosis and categorization—are likely primary considerations.

Those forces influencing or otherwise bringing about handicap may be the most serious for users of human services, and the role expansion inherent in consumerism at least within human service systems can serve as a correction for handicap. It can advance what Wolfensberger (2013). came to call social role valorization. Inherent in the idea of valorization is the enhancement of role and ultimately status. It seeks to counteract diminished status in which people who are marginalized experience a compounding of deviance principally due to the combination of factors, like serious illness and disability that can result from low expectations and opportunities, limited work, and poverty.

Role expansion can open opportunity structures that are too often limited or closed for individuals who are involved in human services, like those coping with the negative societal response to their situations, such as living with serious mental illness or cognitive limitations. Most systems of human services, particularly those adopting a medical model in which the diagnosis and treatment of long-term illness are central to helping, too often fail to incorporate the competencies to address stigma and deviance experienced by those they seek to assist.

The movement to involve recipients of services as peer support specialists within human service systems, especially rehabilitation or mental health systems of care, can use employment within the system in two ways. The system itself can use the employment of peer support specialists as a means to make the supports they offer people more sensitive and responsive. And, the system can use peer support employment as a rehabilitation strategy offering people accommodated employment within a culture in which performance expectations can be managed to facilitate the success of individuals whose record of employment may not be strong.

Role expansion within human service systems can express itself in four ways:

- Opening of work and employment options for recipients helping them use those opportunities as a way of augmenting their experience, success, and social capital.
- Participation in governance at multiple levels of the system including boards of directors and advisory boards. Involvement in shaping the policies of systems of care can enable recipients to expand their sense of efficacy within the system altering interactions between themselves and others who hold more powerful roles within human service systems, like administrators, managers, and supervisors.
- Involvement in evaluation and research activities in which recipients have opportunities to influence the design and implementation of those activities through the introduction of their perspectives and experiences as recipients. The introduction of those perspectives and experiences can alter the relationships of recipients with those who

possess more power. Such alteration in power relationships in which recipients feel more influence over existing arrangements of helping can potentially increase self-efficacy.

- Controlling support systems as an augmentation of care within the existing framework and arrangements of human service systems can further enhance the efficacy recipients can experience. Augmentation here means that the support system operated by and for recipients adds an aspect of care that is of material significance to its members.

Providers of care and recipients should consider the substantive material significance of consumer roles a system incorporates. Is it an important modification of the human service system that augments care in new ways, taps into the strengths of recipients, and uses those strengths to advance the well-being of the population of recipients? Is the modification permanent and is it institutionalized, particularly within the policy structure of the human service system, and within its funding? In this sense, an important consideration here involves the institutionalization of expanded roles the system incorporates.

Part of this institutionalization involves the extent to which human service professionals adopt positive attitudes toward role expansion itself and the incumbents of those roles that reflect the altered status of recipients within the system. The attitudes of those who manage, supervise, and serve as colleagues toward recipients and those who are in empowered roles are central factors in institutionalization. Potentially those actors may raise numerous issues to underscore the limitations of those who occupy consumer roles that are a product of a system's policy of consumer role expansion and status enhancement. They may point out ethical considerations, limitations in knowledge, personal capacities, boundary issues, and problems of expertise. But those criticisms can fail to recognize the distinctive assets recipients as active consumers can bring to human system roles. They can introduce new realities, reveal new procedures or tactics of interaction, augment empathy and sympathetic regard, and expand sensitivity to recipients' situations who are receiving support from their peers.

A central issue in enhancing consumerism within human systems involves its consequences for those recipients who experience role expansion. The recipients' involvement in the innovation can change them considerably, especially in ways people come to think about themselves. Success in roles can facilitate efficacy, which can heighten people's sense of accomplishment, personal confidence, and influence their aims and goals in life. Those actors who are involved in framing and enacting role expansion should remain mindful of these potential changes and prepare themselves for addressing the consequences of such alterations in organizational policy.

Translating these consequences into other opportunities for recipients who have participated in expanded roles is important involving other employment opportunities, new career lines, participation in education, particularly post-secondary education, and transition into statuses as credentialed human service professionals. The latter may be especially important for those individuals who become interested in using their experiences as recipients and consumers as assets and credentials for career progression in the human services. Problematic here is when role expansion is temporary but alters the incumbents' perceptions of themselves and then the innovation comes to an end or is dropped because of lapses in funding.

Consumers unlikely call into question the reality of the issues with which they are dealing. And they likely may not readily critique the arrangements of care they are receiving although assertive consumers, especially highly assertive ones, may face considerable sanction or negative reactions if they pursue an avenue of self-advocacy. Many recipients readily look to professionals as the sources of assistance they want for themselves. For consumers, the principal questions likely involve humanization of themselves as enfranchised individuals, involvement, and influence over treatment, prescriptions for the humanization of a system that can violate people's integrity and trust (O'Brien, 2002). Related here is the achievement of quality of care as well as related properties relevant to service system design including availability, access, appropriateness, and affordability. The achievement of collaboration between service provider and recipient is central to consumerism and its purpose is to humanize the system and personalize care (O'Brien, 2002). Issues pertaining to the scope of choice, the involvement in treatment planning, and the engagement of peer and mutual support distinguish consumerism in human

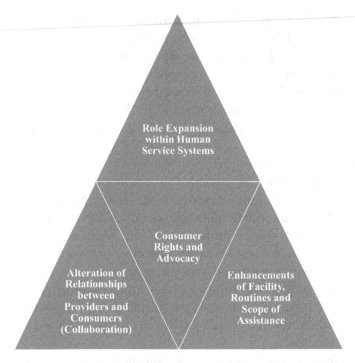

Fig. 3.1 Consumerism as enhanced status of recipients within human service organizations

service systems (Moxley & Mowbray, 1997). Figure 3.1 offers a way of thinking about consumerism involving role expansion within human services. Central here are the enhancements within established systems for humanizing the involvement of consumers.

Survivors and Role Innovation

Those who identify themselves as ex-patients or survivors likely have an adversarial relationship with providers and their organizations or alternatively, they seek to distance themselves from what they see as unwarranted intrusion by various systems. They likely do not see such intrusion as legitimate, that it serves as a form of social control, and that it is inherently abusive. Thus, the establishment of alternative support structures, ones that stand outside of formal systems, is innovative. Such places offer refuge, insulating participants from a society that could exact considerable toll on people's well-being including mood, outlook, and behavior. A larger critique of society, one that induced what the established society defined as mental illness by virtue of the considerable stress it creates, is also a salient element of this movement. This critique serves as a grand narrative of survivorship and it often incorporates themes of societal injustice and oppression of people who experience considerable marginalization (Scheper-Hughes & Lovell, 1986).

Unlike consumers, survivors may question the reality of deviance and thereby bring into question the legitimacy of human service systems. From the vantage of survivors, such systems are seen as part of the structure of social control and, in this way, are no different than any other societal institution that uses oppression as a way of managing what are otherwise diverse forms of cognitive, emotional, behavioral or social diversity, or appearance. Survivors are not interested in advancing the quality of care those systems offer, and, in this way, they are different from those who accept the status of consumer. The development of mutual support systems, however, is important given the proliferation of local support groups and/or alternative organizations survivors create.

One can observe movements to delegitimize professionals in other arenas of human services. Veterans may eschew formal systems of care, especially mental health or substance use care, offered by administrative units of government like the Veterans Administration. Activists may come to see themselves as survivors of the military system and its hegemony over their personal and family lives. They may find solace in support from other veterans who are survivors of the military system. Vietnam veterans organized among themselves in the face of governmental neglect, or disdain by citizens at large who did not valorize their service and even sacrifice.

Support systems may emerge among homeless individuals who eschew formal assistance. They may gather in their own camps and form their own governance in managing their communities. Homeless individuals may demonstrate against the establishment, and confront law enforcement officials who disrupt those camps through the enforcement of vagrancy or loitering laws.

As I have discussed earlier in this monograph, the deaf community has a long history of self-help and mutual support their members created through their affiliation as students enrolled in state schools for the deaf. These support systems form as clubs in which members stay affiliated across their life span oftentimes finding spouses or partners through the members of those clubs. People with disabilities form their own support systems mindful that human service professionals represent oppression they experience by the general society. The protest of ADAPT is a salient example of how support systems can link with social activism in which people with physical disabilities confront the representatives of existing community power structures to demand opportunities, alterations in the physical structure of buildings and communities, and access to vital services like transportation.

These examples are grounded in the experience of inequity. People who do not readily fit into the mainstream, who are different in a world unaccepting of diversity, and who experience outright neglect from established institutions, organize to advance their own interests. Mutual support is a principal resource within such self-organization and the self-help it sets in motion can counteract the neglect people experience from the greater society and its institutions. This neglect and the process of self-organization are the building blocks of a group's narrative of existence and purpose.

The idea of survivorship is central to this narrative. The members likely see themselves as survivors of a greater societal neglect manifest in the members of a particular group forming a "social problem." Survivors are such because they survive the societal response to their situations of discrimination, societal neglect, and marginalization. They survive the professional response to the issues they face, which from the perspective of survivors are more political in nature than products of their deficiencies that the system of response may seek to legitimate. And, survivors may see themselves as having to cope with their own internalization of society's negative labeling processes. In this manner, the factors influencing survivorship are complex. Survivorship forms a sector of support external to formal systems of human services. And, for good reason. Those who are survivors come to learn that investing trust in professionals can create multiple negative consequences.

Survivor organizations are operated "for and by members," and the membership model can be an important element of their cultures. Given a variety of social forces, members are likely sensitive to stress, may not have adequate basic resources to support their independent living, need support to offset isolation, and want a place with which they can affiliate and affirm their identities. Such local organizations, however, are not extensions of a human service system. They form based on dissent. Given such formation they offer members opportunities to withdraw from formal systems and find safety or even sanctuary in group life through which organizations form distinctive cultures, many times based on resistance to the status quo. Innovation becomes a salient quality of these cultures.

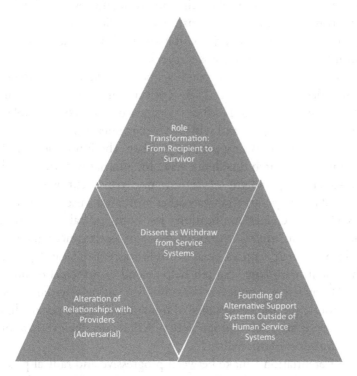

Fig. 3.2 Dissent as a form of consumerism

The organizations themselves can create new roles for members, ones that can carry considerable responsibility, scope of action, and rival those held by professionals.

Figure 3.2 captures the building blocks of consumerism within human services as dissent. The essence of dissent involves people rejecting human services and their ethos in favor of mutual support, self-help, and collective social action.

Cooperation and Conflict

Human service systems, consumerism, and survivorship cleave along an axis of *cooperation* in the case of consumerism and *conflict* in the case of survivorship. For consumers, the system is potentially good and can become more responsive to its recipients through progressive policies of consumerism, particularly as consumers experience considerable role change and, as a consequence, become involved in humanizing a system and improving its responsiveness to peers.

Alternatively, for survivors, conflict may dominate their interactions with providers and officials. Their critical stance on the system can increase social distance, and induce, as a consequence, considerable innovation in mutual support and self-help arrangements outside of a system as survivors organize to support one another. The innovation itself may evolve out of the search dissidents make for alternative forms based on a conflict-oriented paradigm of action, one consistent with resistance reflective of *emancipatory* strategies other movements use within a society.

This cleavage creates implications for both radical and progressive practices. The encompassing critique survivors assert concerning the societal role of human services creates implications for radical practice in which dissent, withdraw, and self-help ascend as principal or dominant values. Alternatively, a policy of consumerism within a system or organization underscores the importance of humanization and personalization, two values that are vital to progressive practice since their realization further legitimizes professionalism.

The differentiation I make between progressive and radical practice is neither nominal nor trivial. They represent two potential grand strategies social human service professionals can pursue in their efforts to operate responsive human service systems or help establish alternative cultures of support.

Factors Differentiating the Identities of Consumers and Survivors

The manner in which I use the idea of culture is consistent with organizational theory. Relevant here is Schein's (2016) treatment of culture as a set of beliefs and values that structure routine. As behavioral patterns crystallize into those routines, members of the entity take them for granted, create norms to govern their consistent use, award and sanction behaviors that deviate from those routines, and create environments, both physical and psychological ones, that support the enactment of those routines. The routines themselves reflect a concretization of behavior, and artifacts emerge to reinforce the culture that forms as a "taken for granted" property of life. The culture itself guides the selection of members and those who remain and those who leave influence the further formation of culture. The idea of membership demographics is important here since the qualities of people that a culture attracts and those who remain, particularly in the long run, further shape and reinforce organizational life.

Culture does not stand alone, however, in facilitating our understanding of the consumerist elements of contemporary human service systems or those survivalist entities that stand apart from those systems. Institutionalization factors into the formation of the various cultures of consumerism. Consistent with Selznick's (2011) thinking about the role of organizations as social institutions in society, each of the options I offer in Chap. 4 incorporates a distinctive set of values, ones that are precarious since members can easily compromise them or those outside of an organization can vitiate them.

Imagine the founding and subsequent development of an innovative ex-patient organization. It is dedicated to enacting a critical assessment of prevailing mental health programs within a given community, stands as an adversary of the mental health system as a whole, and seeks to demonstrate new ways of supporting people who are marginalized by pejorative mental health labeling as a tool of social control. The entity incorporates the arts and performance strategies as a vehicle for operationalizing its critical values in action and with the voluntary involvement of members the organization delivers what it calls "critical consciousness raising" performances throughout the community, frequently undertaking these in a style of delivery involving spontaneous and improvised events (such as the engagement in poetry critical of mental health programs) in public areas.

Founded some two decades ago by a charismatic ex-patient leader, the entity struggles with resources, and after rejecting numerous offers of funding by the existing mental health system the organization remains separate from the organized mental health system even though it offers support to some 500 people annually. But even with uncertain funding, the entity has crystallized into an organization, obtains minor amounts of resources from foundation and community arts sources, and is led by a strong lay board of people who have had negative experiences with the mental health system. Independent of two members who bring financial expertise to the governance of the organization, composing the board are members who consider themselves ex-patients or survivors.

The critical stance the organization incorporates is indeed precarious and its distancing from the established mental health system, its engagement in the arts as a tool of critical consciousness, and its socialization of members into adversarial relationships with dominant mental health administrators serve as principal tactics reflective of its essential values. Offers of funding by the dominant mental health system reflect the precarious nature of the values the organization embraces.

For Selznick, the dominant mental health system is engaging in a form of co-optation. It is seeking to gain control over an entity that challenges the mental health system but is in a less powerful position. This form of co-optation makes the institutionalization of the ex-survivor entity even more precarious. But in this case the organization's assertion of its core values and its own continuity as a community entity demonstrates its achievement of integrity. For the most part, it adheres to its core values, protects them, uses them to create and deploy strategies, employs them in a manner that affirms its identity as an organization dedicated to the support of ex-patients, and engages them in a program of dissent.

Conclusion

I raise this example not only to illuminate the dynamics of institutionalization but also to consider how each type I offer in the following chapter is precarious given the nature of what it represents as an expression of a particular response to professional hegemony within a given community, when the central character of that care is social control. Each type I offer next incorporates a certain kind of ideology, a set of ideas that fuel its belief systems, and a distinctive culture.

Earlier in this chapter I identify two dominant ideologies, each formed by how people come to define their relationship with the existing social institution of human services within a given community. The consumerist ideology legitimates both the reality of problematic behavior seen through a professional lens and the necessity of a sound response from a human service system. This ideology likely embraces the prevailing paradigms about both the causes of human deviance and desirable ways of managing it within systems of professional intervention.

Alternatively, the ex-patient ideology likely embraces a political perspective on who a community seeks to control, and the manner in which a community seeks to manage a particular group. Basically, this ideology embraces ideas pertaining to oppression, social control, and marginalization as intentional strategies a community (or society) uses to manage those it deems inappropriate, bothersome, problematic, undesirable, or dangerous.

References

Mowbray, C., Moxley, D., Jasper, C., & Howell, L. (Eds.). (1997). *Consumers as providers in psychiatric rehabilitation*. IAPSRS.

Mowbray, C., Moxley, D., & Van Tosh, L. (2001, May). Changing roles for primary consumers in community psychiatry. In J. Talbot & R. Hales (Eds.),

Textbook of administrative psychiatry: New concepts for a changing behavioral health system (2nd ed.). American Psychiatric Publishing, Inc..

Moxley, D. P., & Mowbray, C. T. (1997, April). Consumers as providers: Social forces and factors legitimizing role innovation in psychiatric rehabilitation. In C. T. Mowbray, D. Moxley, C. Jasper, & L. Davis (Eds.), *Consumers as providers in psychiatric rehabilitation*. International Association of Psychosocial Rehabilitation Services.

O'Brien, J. (2002). Person-centered planning as a contributing factor in organizational and social change. *Research and Practice in Persistent and Severe Disability, 27*, 261–264.

Schein, E. (with Peter Schein) (2016). *Organizational leadership and culture* (5th ed.). Wiley.

Scheper-Hughes, N., & Lovell, A. M. (1986). Breaking the circuit of social control: Lessons in public psychiatry from Italy and Franco Basaglia. *Social Science and Medicine, 23*, 159–178.

Selznick, P. (2011). Leadership in administration. Quid Pro.

Wolfensberger, W. (2013). A brief introduction to social role valorization. Valor Press.

4

Typology of Consumerism and Survivorship

Introduction

How can we come to appreciate the types of consumerism and how they manifest themselves in diverse statuses and roles within systems of human services, or outside of human services (a distinction of which serves as the focus of Chap. 6, the inside-outside dimension)? The typology I offer in Fig. 4.1 captures this diversity in status and role within the context of four kinds of consumer cultures. Two axes form those four cultures involving whether (and the extent to which) recipients control outcomes, in other words, what they seek for themselves through their roles, and involving whether recipients control the key processes of the helping or assistance they receive (what I call processes in Fig. 4.1).

I invoke the term recipient in this typology with some hesitation. It serves as an alternative to the concept of client, which too often can be pejorative, with its double meaning for client in ancient Greek life referred to that person who was dependent, typically on a patron, or in certain forms of professional interaction, such as law, in which a person seeks out a lawyer for the purposes of gaining direct assistance. Client in social or human services suggests that the person is often assigned a

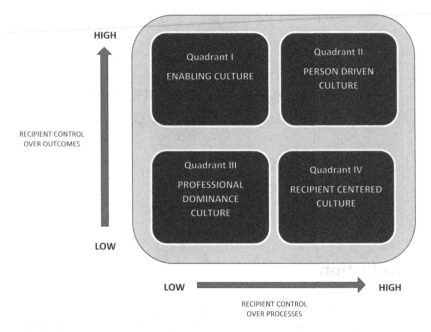

HIGH

RECIPIENT CONTROL
OVER OUTCOMES

LOW

Quadrant I

ENABLING CULTURE

Quadrant II

PERSON DRIVEN
CULTURE

Quadrant III

PROFESSIONAL
DOMINANCE
CULTURE

Quadrant IV

RECIPIENT CENTERED
CULTURE

LOW   HIGH

RECIPIENT CONTROL
OVER PROCESSES

Fig. 4.1 A typology of four cultures

worker because of a determination of need outside of their ability to fulfill it directly. And, often, some representative of society determines that need and invokes the helping process for that person.

Consumerism or survivorship takes the recipient status to a higher level of choice and control. Expressed in multiple roles in relationship to human services, consumerism suggests that the person who experiences a need has some control over what they want for themselves. They have power to determine that need and they may control the resources to create the relationships or situations they wish for themselves. This kind of control or personal agency can serve as a form of empowerment in human services.

Four Alternatives of Consumerism

Figure 4.1 serves as a heuristic to order contemporary human services into the four quadrants visible within the figure. Certainly, there are other possibilities, but these four quadrants emerge out of the extent to which recipient control over ends and means intersect to create distinctive cultures. I treat the quadrants themselves as cultures in which beliefs and values as well as artifacts coalesce into a distinctive type of helping or assistance. Within each culture a certain configuration of consumer status or role emerges revealing the diversity in which consumerism can manifest itself in those structures that constitute human services.

For sure, the figure is a simplification but like any typology it seeks to portray the essence of an entity, which in this case manifests itself as a human service organization or whole system. That system in its totality can encapsulate people who do not quite fit into the mainstream of society. How society relates to those individuals, those who do not fit into mainstream values the greater society prescribes to define normativity, or who may violate those values, legitimate the existence of human service organizations or systems.

So, the typology incorporates two principal dimensions both of which vary from low to high. The dimensions are continuous since while their orthogonality communicates some independence their intersection form four pure types while different degrees of them implicate the possibility that hybrids exist within contemporary human services.

Liberalization of a given system can occur for the purposes of legitimization of human services as a dominant part of a society's social welfare institution. The system itself may introduce consumerism to restructure the relationships between recipients and helping professionals. Consumerism may serve as a tactic for relaxing or inhibiting the power of what can be dominant professionals who can control the direction a particular group of people can assume, or influence quite dramatically the life opportunities among those particular people. Ultimately, however, the power of professionals remains in such arrangements and indeed can be well entrenched within human service systems engaging in such liberalization.

Quadrants III and IV represent such liberalization when the consumerist ideology of human service leaders or practitioners endorse either a heightened form of professional dominance as in Quadrant III or as in Quadrant IV relax that dominance to focus on bringing recipients into the mainstream of those forums in which they can contribute to decisions about how to structure the supports they want for themselves. These quadrants suggest cultures in which recipients as consumers do not actually control the direction their support takes. In other words, they do not really specify the outcomes they want since such specification likely remains with the professionals who control the rules of interaction, those that flow from the ultimate policies of the system itself.

If Quadrants III and IV represent liberalization in which new role packages of recipients emerge in the form of internal consumerism, Quadrants I and II heighten the control of recipients over the ends of human services, that is what they want for themselves even if they do not control key processes (such as in Quadrant I) or control those processes and the outcomes they should produce. Those two quadrants reflect true empowerment within human services, and influence not only the role packages of consumers (or survivors) but those of professionals as well. Indeed, Quadrant II brings into question whether professionals are actually even needed as primary providers of assistance. Alternatively, Quadrant I suggests that the professional is instrumental in helping consumers define their direction but the professional may then undertake the process of helping on their own to achieve the outcomes consumers want, but who may lack the expertise to control the process of assistance. Here consumers do not have the expertise they need to resolve the issues they define as problematic.

The Organization of Human Services

The regions of the figure itself conceptually form a whole that constitutes how human service systems (inclusive of their policies, funding, paradigms, models, organizations, personnel, and participants) structure themselves in relationship to societal purpose. Each quadrant suggests a particular societal purpose I summarize as follows:

- Quadrant I: Society possesses an interest in an empowered person who achieves what they want for themselves through the agency of a professional who has the power and standing to confront social institutions diminishing the consumer's status, or limiting their scope of action.
- Quadrant II: The person should exercise their own agency, particularly in concert with people who share similar circumstances, and although society may establish resource systems to facilitate such mutual support and self-help, it is best that society itself minimizes its intrusion into the lives of those individuals.
- Quadrant III: Through either their vulnerability or dependency, or the potential danger a person's character, conduct and/or behavior present, society has a real interest in protecting the person and other members of society from that person through empowered professionals whose decision-making and action are dominant within formal human service systems.
- Quadrant IV: Society has an interest in an active recipient whose participation can influence their subsequent recovery and the restoration or development of their civic virtue and social responsibility.

Horizontal Axis of the Typology

The horizontal dimension reflects the degree to which recipients in the case of consumers or participants in alternatives in which they possess control over the support they offer and receive. Support is an essential dimension here for its well-documented influence on well-being and social functioning. Whether a person identifies as a consumer or ex-patient, isolation takes its toll on a person's outlook, mood, cognition, and effective coping with the challenges and exigencies of daily life. My assumption is that social support, in its many forms, and diversities, is an essential element of health and well-being. The horizontal axis incorporates this vital dimension of human well-being.

Vertical Axis of the Typology

The vertical dimension addresses the control recipients or participants exercise over the outcomes the helping effort produces involving the opportunities recipients or participants have for specifying those outcomes, and in prioritizing what they seek to achieve for themselves. The potential outcome space within human services or community development (in the case of survivors) is quite broad, particularly when a conceptual framework of quality of life shapes the contours of this space, although the potential scope of outcome can be substantially narrowed through the adoption of a medicalized theory of action.

Narrowing of the outcome space may occur through the determination of medical necessity, and implicating the control of symptoms in the domains of cognition, affect, and behavior in service to the achievement of some semblance of normative behavior often manifest in social role functioning. Indeed, whether the human service form expresses itself in medical care, rehabilitation, or community support the achievement of normative behavior and related social role functioning may be the aims guiding human services.

The outcome set governing those alternatives in which participants are active in creating their own support systems may be more fluid and flexible, and they may be quite broad focusing on the support of the person and the enhancement of the person's status through augmentation of social services, legal assistance, and social action. Outcomes within such alternatives may encompass something as simple as a felt sense of safety but also extend into domains fundamental to the achievement of quality of life such as culture, work, education, business, and housing development.

The Typology as a Whole

The typology refrains from prescribing the kinds of support or outcomes a system should produce. It is configured to capture the perspective of the person who is the participant in the system, and the principal value the typology incorporates is the degree of real or perceived control the person exercises within each type. Personal control itself may be one of the most fundamental properties of a system culture, and it is something both a medical and negative social reaction may diminish for people who experience a label of deviance and the associated stigma such labeling can produce.

The conceptual nature of the typology may very well obscure how actual consumer or ex-patient options operate within or outside any given system. Some options may possess either consumerist or ex-patient images in name only. The system may be quite adept in co-opting those options and putting them to use so as to reinforce the integrity of care devoted to the medicalization of deviance, which may stand as either an explicit or latent strategic objective of a particular system of care. The consumerist options the system offers may not be central in this regards and are ancillary or complementary to medical management.

Moving away from the cells of the typology, and viewing the actual vectors, one can observe how Quadrants I and III depend on professionals either to control situations as in Quadrant III or as advocates, as in Quadrant I. Alternatively, Quadrants II and IV assume an active participant to make each type operate in practice. Still, Quadrants I and II likely are the most empowerment-oriented options since theoretically people control the principal aims of action. Quadrants III and IV are treatment-oriented. Here recipients participate in treatment, rehabilitation, or person change efforts under the host of professionals.

Conclusion: A Hybrid Example

I have observed systems of care in which medicalization is ancillary or complementary to strategies of peer support and personal development of recipients. In one case an entity, which the author refers to as Concord, a pseudonym, serving people identified as having serious mental illness occupied a former warehouse that was subdivided into employment, housing, and cultural development zones. Dominating the anterior portion of the building was a café open to members and workers from local businesses who dined at the small restaurant during lunch or who patronized the café for takeout cuisine. I invoke the term cuisine purposively since the organization was known in the community more for its lunch options than as a support system for people with serious mental illness.

When touring the building, I found it difficult programmatically and architecturally to discern the location of psychiatric treatment and medical care. As Schein (2016) notes, such arrangements are easy to observe but difficult to interpret. When I inquired into the whereabouts of this programmatic option, the tour guide led me to an exterior building, humble and small, which housed the offices of a psychiatrist, psychiatric social worker, and nurse.

This exemplar reveals the danger of treating the contents of Fig. 4.1 as fixed and inflexible options. The types do serve as a heuristic for dialogue, and can stimulate reflection informing organizational development and program design. Concord is instructive here. Participants in Concord were not patients. They were members. Some were chefs and others were culinary professionals in training. Concord affirmed the existence of serious mental illness as a bona fide medical category necessitating medical management but that conception was not central to daily operations. Concord's members accepted such a diagnostic stance as necessary but ancillary.

Medical management was subordinated to the personal development of a Concord member who could receive continuous support in key areas of quality of life, especially cultural development (through the arts; Feen-Calligan et al., 2009), employment (through a member-run business), vocational development (learning to engage in kitchen work and food preparation), and housing that Concord controlled itself and made available to its members.

Concord is an example of a hybrid entity encompassing qualities of several types, particularly those that I label as enabling and recipient-centered cultures. However, the dominant type defines the character of this entity as a recipient-centered culture. In the case of Concord, normalization comes to pervade the organization. That participants are productive members of the community, and their serious mental illness is subordinate to the rehabilitative features of the program, means for me that the entity comes to be seen as a normal part of the larger local community. Its facility fits into the surroundings, and Concord may be more a culinary option within the community than a rehabilitative one. Ambiguity of intent may be one of Concord's principal organizational strengths.

Here too the organization lays the foundation of social role valorization. Members engage in roles that are central to community life. Media coverage valorizes the participants as culinary artists who create meals for members of the local community, especially the business community. For Wolfensberger, who coined the idea of social role valorization, deviance fades in its salience as people are seen as occupying critical roles within the greater community. Here too the idea of the competence-deviance hypothesis is operative. According to Gold, the hypothesis sets the stage for mastery and competence and how they produce social standing within a given community. The members of Concord can master individually or co-produce within group life the culinary arts along with other forms of artistic performance including music, theater, and the visual arts.

Ultimately, the organizational form Concord assumes in the human services is quite interesting. Concord is a principal asset within its local community. The organization and its members contribute a great deal to the quality of day, quality of life, and standard of living of the local community. Concord's role as an organizational citizen within the community is an important one and the individuals who are active members make important contributions underscoring their civic virtue. Aggregated across individuals, the social purpose of Concord heightens the standing of its social productivity.

Some may be rightfully critical of this kind of hybrid. Close inspection suggests that Concord incorporates a human resource approach to rehabilitation rather than a medical one. People learn about and explore roles and learn about the demands of those roles by contributing to a greater social purpose, and by building identities as workers. That the psychiatric model is present but of limited status indicates to me that it serves a handmaiden role within the organization. Psychiatric professionals work in the background and facilitate members' involvement in the life of the organizational community of Concord. By handmaiden, I mean that the psychiatric model serves a secondary function within the organizational community. Thus, as a hybrid, Concord incorporates a limited form of professional dominance as it prioritizes all of the virtues of a broadened scope of recipient participation. The recipient-centered culture, therefore, is apparent. Members' involvement in a work-ordered day is a principal focus of rehabilitation, and it is up to members to engage in those processes of rehabilitation as they pursue the outcome set Concord sets for the membership.

The incorporation of the arts, whether performing, visual, or culinary, is a means to activate the full development of a person who through their membership can come to appreciate their talents, interests, and achievements in concrete ways. The alignment of physical health activities, such as through a health-based psychiatry, with creative endeavors that reaches a market in the case of the culinary productivity of Concord, is a testimony to the ultimate normalization aims this facility seeks to realize with its participants or members.

References

Feen-Calligan, H., Washington, O., & Moxley, D. P. (2009). Homelessness among older African American women: Interpreting a serious social issue through the arts in community based participatory action research. *New Solutions: Journal of Environmental and Occupational Health Policy, 19*(4), 423–448.

Schein, E. (with Peter Schein) (2016). *Organizational leadership and culture* (5th ed.). Wiley.

5

Cultures of Consumerism in Human Services

Introduction

Figure 4.1 incorporates four pure types of consumerism that serve heuristic purposes. The validity of the typology extends from my experience garnered through several decades of action research to document expressions of those types through a variety of technical assistance, consultation, and organizational development projects. The four cultures encompass considerable diversity in organizational culture and form, but invite further conceptualization and criticism. Most of all, they challenge a principal question of importance to either progressive or radical work in the human services. That is, what constitutes a human service system?

Today, as an outcome of movements the aim of which is the humanization of social institutions, and the emergence of multiple strategies of human services, yet another question gains prominence: what constitutes a contemporary human service system defined principally by its adherents and its dissidents? Each of the following types illuminates an aspect of this question that I address more fully in the conclusion of this chapter. However, in this chapter, I engage each of the four types as cultures.

© The Author(s), under exclusive license to Springer Nature Singapore Pte Ltd. 2021
D. P. Moxley, *Consumerism in the Human Services*,
https://doi.org/10.1007/978-981-16-7192-0_5

The Idea of Culture

I invoke the idea of culture to capture beliefs and values about people's status and roles within a given society or, in this chapter, within a particular system of human services. Emanating from statuses and roles are opportunities a system allocates based on perceived necessities or the merit and worth the system attaches to those statuses and roles. Within the monograph, I have used the concept of diminished status in which a society purposefully strips from people or groups life-sustaining necessities or life-enhancing opportunities. The differential allocation of status and roles and the opportunities adhering to them implicates oppression a society can exert through the purposeful enactment of discrimination and stigma. Prejudice can animate these social dynamics further justifying what amounts to systemic abuse. By systemic, I am referring to those cultures a society creates to manage certain groups of people in ways that diminish their quality of life, and their well-being.

The manifest expression of these societal dynamics can be found in marginalization. The society and its institutions push people to the periphery of the society and degrade their quality of life. The society can deprive groups of health-producing circumstances and degrade food, air, soil, housing, physical and spatial qualities and then (paradoxically) burden those who experience such circumstances with the responsibility for being in the situation that a society creates. Why does this occur? Because of the root issue inherent in discrimination and prejudice and what flows from these: oppression that serves a social management purpose.

Too often human service systems reflect the greater societal dynamics producing marginalization. In Chap. 7, I offer the concept of human management as a product of societal culture, that is, its basic beliefs concerning human merit and worth. That I offer such logic implicates the political nature of human services when those systems produce human management models that degrade people's lives or uplift those lives. In Chap. 7, I address the negative models of human management, as well as positive ones. A system's adaption to the belief system of the greater society, or a system's engagement in creating alternative cultures, influences its human management models.

Still people who bear the negative effects the greater society and its culture produce can organize themselves building systems of support under their own control and establishing their own routines, procedures, practices, and policies. It is those qualities that form the manifest expression of cultures under the control of members. Such cultures, according to Douglas and Nye (1998), involve cohesive groups in which members organize around weak structures. Those groups may turn on the self-actualization of their members and the creation of capabilities among members to fulfill their needs.

Human management models likely have architectures, temporal qualities, locations, and resources that form from either a system's adaptation to the prevailing culture or its rejection of that culture. Indeed, as I consider each of the four cultures, I offer systemic cultures of adaptation—when the system itself accepts the prevailing view of a person who experiences marginalization or rejection when the response seeks to distance itself from the prevailing paradigm. Paradigm likely flows from adaptation to or rejection of the prevailing culture.

Paradigm raises questions in my mind about whether cultures of human services can actually innovate in relationship to consumer status and role as this occurs within a given system (see Chap. 6 as I make a distinction between consumerism inside and outside of a human service system). No matter how established human service systems differ, they may share a common paradigm of how they define and adapt to a particular social issue. My subsequent discussion of Wiseman's videography raises an interesting question about the durability of paradigm within human services.

Archetypes influence the formation of paradigms since they offer a deeply seeded set of perceptions of what constitutes deviance. Distinctive responses can crystallize around those archetypes yielding forms like incarceration, torture, geographic degradation, or community management. Archetypes can be either positive or negative, but negative ones are likely if a society seeks to defend itself from those who may be seen as threatening the status quo, a threat that may be visible in the violation of a society's standards of purity. A defensive society may likely possess strong boundaries delimiting who is within or outside of the mainstream—that is, who is included and who is excluded. A society that is well bounded may treat people harshly or benevolently, but what those strategies share in common is the purposeful management of those who differ in various ways from what the society defines as meritorious and worthy. The allocation of roles and statuses may occur in such well-bounded systems to communicate across group lines those values the society prioritizes and enforces.

The Types as Cultures

The Culture of Professional Dominance and Control

Within this culture, the medicalization of social ills tends to be dominant if not controlling. Medicalization and related disease management involving issues of self-care, professional oversight, and case management are defining attributes of the culture. Consistent with the societal movement of managed care with its emphasis on efficiency, contemporary human service systems have incorporated medical explanations and narratives concerning the genetic, biological, and psychosocial aspects of human problems. Within the framework I offer in Fig. 4.1, within organizational or program cultures in which professional dominance is the principal defining attribute, recipient control over either processes of support or outcomes is low, nonexistent, and/or nominal. This absence of control means that recipients have limited influence over the process of their care and management may become a principal systems value.

The rationalization of human management is a principal cultural aim of this type such that there are established protocols guiding the provision of physical, cognitive, and psychosocial management of people whom the greater society may see as unfit in the achievement of social integration or inclusion. Adherence is a principal outcome of this type since symptom management often at a behavioral level is an important part of the equation of care.

The involvement of highly credentialed individuals led by professionals with advanced degrees often organized in team structures where there is involvement of other professionals who hold specialized roles within the system of care is also a salient element of this culture. Those professionals can include psychologists, nurses, counselors, social workers, and rehabilitation personnel, such as occupational therapists. A collaborative value may link those professionals into cross-functional teams the members of which coordinate care. And, credentialing, certification, licensure, and accreditation may be dominant system management tools ensuring that the system itself adheres to professionalization.

Supplementing this team may be a navigation capacity that facilitates the movement of the recipient (or patient) through a rationalized system of care that is designed to facilitate the treatment process and the achievement of outcomes relevant to human management. Navigators may be highly trained and credentialed professionals, such as nurses, or they may involve non-credentialed workers who have expertise formed through their direct experience with the human problem the system is designed to address, such as physical disability.

Navigators within complex systems of human management can involve peer support specialists who work directly with recipients/patients to help them achieve continuity of care, a property important to the integrity of this culture. Navigators may be cultural too. They can work with professionals in navigating cultural situations enabling those professionals to interact with other groups of which they are not members or readily accepted. Cultural liaisons can interpret professional actions to their peers, and bring language skills to situations that professionals may not possess. Alternatively, they can enable professionals to better understand the culture of people who are potential or actual recipients.

The criticism of medical or professional dominance has a long-standing focus within the social sciences, cultural criticism, psychosocial helping professions, journalism, and film. This criticism harkens back to the critique of medical hegemony, the disavowal of social responsibility for people who face serious deprivation, and the horrific conditions operating within total institutions. The critical response of ex-patients to this hegemony remains a potent force in shaping the rights of people whose deprivation the society produces either through acts of omission or through those of commission.

Yet contemporary criticism of existing human service arrangements that incorporate professional dominance do not necessarily bring into question the legitimacy of human management itself, but often raises issues about coverage, accessibility, appropriateness, and adequacy of that management. Increasingly there is a call for the involvement of professionals in the prevention and management of high-risk situations, such as ones involving individuals with mental health backgrounds who engage in spree killings using automatic weapons (Stern, 2012; Viebeck, 2012). Strengthening the legitimacy of a medical view of mental health concerns are efforts to integrate primary health care and mental health, augment the primary health care of people labeled as seriously mentally ill, and the pervasive use of disease management protocols. Still movements focusing on the integration of human services into medical management, and a broadened framework of what constitutes health, can incorporate substance use treatment, behavioral management, and the management of cognition. Coordination among professionals solidify their instrumentality. Integration across domains of human problems densify organizations and interorganizational networks.

The Enabling Culture: Professional Facilitation for Issue Resolution

The enabling culture incorporates those entities that facilitate the achievement of client-defined goals through processes, activities, and forms of support offered by professionals working independently of the recipient but on their behalf. The culture of this alternative is based on a belief that people coping with deprivation face considerable stigma and marginalization. This stigma creates needs that go unmet, erects organizational barriers to the fulfillment of those needs, and produces numerous issues that can further exacerbate societally induced symptoms, including anxiety, hostility, depression, frustration, and demoralization. And, unresolved needs, particularly those that threaten survival, may create considerable distress that interferes with social role functioning.

Society may channel such individuals into narrow benefit structures, and then ration the availability of these benefits, or place them under bureaucratic management incorporating rigid rule systems. It likely takes a seasoned professional to help individuals seeking benefits to decipher the system, make appeals, and sustain action over time. Such action likely constitutes advocacy within or outside of human service or benefits systems.

Professionals within and outside human services systems fulfill roles as representatives of individuals coping with considerable unfulfilled need, through which they address the social consequences labeling enacts, particularly stigma. As representative, the professional works with recipients to help them define the issues they face and the outcomes they desire. Or, recipients may bring to those professionals' clear conceptions of outcomes they want to bring about. Recipients may simply be without the motivation or energy as well as the networks, know-how, and expertise to undertake sustained action to bring about the outcomes they seek.

The enabling culture allows recipients to relinquish control over the process of bringing about the outcomes they desire to the professionals who have the specialized expertise and organizational social capital to bring about the desired ends. Those professionals may work independently of recipients touching base with them to make further decisions about the achievement of outcomes and the reformulation of strategy.

The idea of enabling as a strategy is not negative here. Oftentimes, human service professionals may see enabling as those actions people take to sustain a person's problematic behavior, thereby reinforcing dysfunctional conduct. Alternatively, a positive frame of enabling involves a professional in helping a person within a complex bureaucratic maze to negotiate barriers and impediments to getting what they seek for themselves.

This form of professional representation is prevalent in rights protection and advocacy systems in which professionals use legal or quasi-legal strategies to address issues that recipients introduce. Case management systems may form to address and resolve benefit and quality-of-life issues recipients present. And some forms of guardianship also may operate within enabling cultures (Moxley & Paul, 2005).

Within such culture, the identification, assessment, and framing of issues to resolve and thereby either bring about a desired disposition of those issues or produce a desired outcome differentiate it from the medicalized human management model inherent in the culture of professional dominance. Issues emerge from the status of the person created by the application of the label of disease, illness, inadequacy, or dysfunction. Relieving the distress people experience may be a principal effect of such a culture, and the ensuing improvement in standard of living, quality of environment, and quality of life may reduce symptoms that can trigger acute episodes and result in setbacks.

The alignment of representatives with the interests of recipients imbues this culture with the qualities of advocacy and empowerment. Unlike the professional dominance culture, in which highly credentialed professionals define and prioritize recipient needs, those professionals operating within this culture assign great importance to the issues recipients identify as frustrating or problematic. How the rigid rule structures can produce inordinate distress for a person becomes the focus of enabling. The assistance recipients receive helps them refine their formulation of issues, prioritize them, and define outcomes. Getting to those outcomes is the duty of the professional.

Peer support specialists or other kinds of advocates may serve an important role in such a culture. Their expertise (emanating from their personal experience with deprivation, stigma, marginalization, and impaired organizational responses) can make them effective representatives of people who often are isolated and alone. The intent here is to further humanize enabling culture, reduce the social distance between the representative and recipient, and tap into the experiential knowledge base peer support specialists offer.

But there is a potential alternative here. Alternative forms of advocacy may emerge in which survivors serve as representatives of recipients who lack either the sustaining power or expertise to resolve the issues they face. Those survivors may offer expertise in alternative dispute resolution, quasi-legal representation, or lay advocacy that is adversarial in its orientation. Buttressing representation by ex-patients or survivors may be credentialed attorneys, law clinics associated with university schools of law, and citizen advocacy projects in which volunteers serve as lay advocates to people they consider disadvantaged. Of course, those options may supplement client representation programs in which there is little if any innovation in consumer roles.

The Recipient-Centered Culture of Broad-Based Support

This culture brings support under control of recipients while the ends of the human service system endure outside of their control. Recipient-centered cultures are focused on meeting the essential needs of those people who experience considerable marginalization. They are on-going support systems that are well structured and designed explicitly to fulfill participants' needs for nurturance and affiliation, personalize participants, support personal development, and offer access to life-sustaining resources like food and nutrition, housing, and work. Recipient-centered cultures are prevalent within mental health systems, such as consumer-operated drop-in-centers, consumer-operated businesses, and supported employment or supported education programs. Some are seen as independent of mental health systems, such as clubhouses, and operate as support systems fostering their own identities, facilities, and governance.

Clubhouses are a good case in point of how consumerism has evolved within the mental health domain. Early precursors of clubhouses involved ex-patient groups (here ex-patient meant a person who had left hospital treatment) and in-patient clubs. Evolving out of a peer support group that came together out of necessity for the survival of people with serious mental illness, Fountain House has served as the iconic model of the clubhouse that has achieved considerable diffusion across the world. *Action for Mental Health*, a report published in 1961 by the Joint Commission on Mental Illness and Health, asserted the need for professional involvement in operating consumer initiatives. The emergence of psychiatric rehabilitation as an interdisciplinary field also affirmed consumerism and legitimized the relevance of consumer self-help and peer support.

Both clubhouses and psychiatric rehabilitation centers have emerged as distinctive models of consumerism. They both affirm the reality of mental illness, implement group-oriented social support as tactics to off-set the negative consequences of mental illness, and facilitate social integration through the emphasis they place on vocational development, housing access, cultural involvement, and employment.

The clubhouse mobilizes the healing effects of group cohesion to promote sound decision-making, a work-ordered day, and productive activity among members. Within the clubhouse belief system, these strategies offset the propensity of people with serious mental illness to lapse into isolation, become unproductive, and become inactive. Group life engages members in productive activities in collaboration with peers and staff.

The social architecture of the clubhouse decreases social distance among helpers and members, requires the involvement of members in productive activity by minimizing the number of staff members who work in the clubhouse, and creates small work environments supporting productive activities. From my experience, clubhouses are designed to facilitate vocational development and independent living among people with serious mental illness through social support in small groups, the prevention or resolution of the problems of daily living, and a form of positive surveillance of the health and well-being of members.

Some may feel that my use of surveillance is too strong a word. But within clubhouses surveillance or monitoring, particularly in the form of outreach, is a natural process of keeping track of people who can experience very negative events in their daily lives, become isolated, and find themselves in harm's way, particularly as victims of crime and violence (Teplin et al., 2005). The kind of surveillance I have witnessed actually constitutes a form of caring about people whose involvement in group life can easily fade away. Membership strengthens this caring since people become known for their distinctive personalities and personal qualities rather than by diagnostic stereotypes.

Clubhouse charters prohibit the delivery of formal mental health services, thereby preserving values of peer social support and mutual assistance. Members access formal mental health services through community sources. The clubhouse, however, uses instrumental capacities to facilitate the fulfillment of human needs readily compromised by the primary psychiatric consequences of mental illness as well as by the issues social reaction can produce. Through clubhouse membership, participants can access housing, employment, transportation, and cultural development through cultures that mediate between the member and the greater community. Cohesive group life is a building block of clubhouse culture.

The community becomes a source of those essential resources and the clubhouse can be the portal that facilitates their discovery and use. As people acquire those resources and fulfill their needs, the clubhouse itself can serve as a support system in which people can receive on-going support to sustain and improve their quality of life and independence. The clubhouse, therefore, operates on the logic of group work and exemplifies consumerism for its emphasis on mutual support among peers is a central quality of the model.

The Person-Driven Culture of Self Determination

The person-driven culture is a stark contrast to the other three cultures. It offers a belief system that respects the autonomy of decision-making of the individual, and it affirms the ultimate independence of the individual in the face of institutional, bureaucratic, and professional power (Moxley & Freddolino, 1990, 1994). This culture offers individuals coping with the fall out of societal reaction to their qualities with as much choice as possible. Here within this quadrant, we find patient-initiated innovations like medication-free clinics, ones that rely on psychosocial support, alternative healing methods, affiliative strategies, and stress reduction, as viable alternatives to traditional psychiatric care. And, here we find ex-patient alternatives that reject the hegemony of professional power and the legitimacy of human service systems.

Within this culture, the integrity of the person is paramount emphasizing values like justice and equity in the face of oppression and marginalization. A greater narrative may define within this culture the reality that pejorative labels mask other social issues like oppression emanating out of poverty, displacement, and diminished status created when people do not cooperate with the prevailing normative standards of performance or otherwise accept or enact prevailing standards of success.

The backdrop to this culture reminds us that total institutions served in nineteenth-century America and Europe as a way of managing social issues emerging from immigration and urbanization in which people who did not readily "fit in" were seen as disorganized, failing to adhere to what elites considered as civic virtue. Violation of civic virtue is an important factor here: many societies value self-control and self-directed behavior, and the violation of such values could be easily interpreted as the absence of competence. With a societal emphasis on conformity and social performance, it is easy to see how human service professionals could enforce such norms, and use order and rigid routines within institutions to enforce moral treatment (Bockhoven, 1956).

There is yet another interesting argument here that plays off of the value of equality. If serious mental illness, for example, is a bona vide illness, then from a medical perspective why shouldn't it be treated like any other physical illness? People coping with other medical concerns like epilepsy or diabetes often report a social stigma and negative social reaction to their situations. But such stigma is likely nowhere as strong than it is with serious mental illness.

What society interprets as serious mental illness stands along with the other cognitive disorders (like dementia) in its threat to established values within the greater culture. Laypeople can easily interpret the irregularities in thinking, emotion, and behavior as threats to their safety, as a state of danger. What is interpreted as disordered behavior introduces unpredictability in how to understand a person's conduct. The narrow normative spaces in which only a certain constellation of behavior is found socially acceptable or normal make those who carry pejorative labels stand out in contrast to normative behavioral forms. While they may be seen as potentially violent, it is more likely that people who are so labeled in negative ways are more likely the victims of mistreatment rather than its perpetrators.

The person-centered alternative does not dismiss or minimize vulnerability. But its adherents argue that professional dominance within organized systems creates or otherwise accentuates vulnerability. The options that emerge may remove or seek to obviate this vulnerability and create support systems outside of formal human services and under the direct control of people who consider themselves survivors. Those support systems strive for equity—by correcting for the experience of abuse or neglect or deprivation through the creation of supports under member control. Yet another value, equality, can remove the kind of hierarchy that too frequently characterizes human service systems.

This ideal expresses itself through broad-based participation, control over the purpose and agenda of support, and the realization of outcomes members establish for themselves. Governance of such options is undertaken for and by members without others, such as those from a human service system, enforcing a set of values that members may find intolerable. The value of collectivism inherent in such alternatives may express itself through innovative arrangements that play off of the mechanisms of self-help.

Such alternatives like social enterprises, businesses and co-operatives, cultural development enterprises that incorporate the arts and performance, and intentional community can facilitate social support, nurture identity formation, and catalyze social activism that members may direct toward the criticism of established human service systems (Washington & Moxley, 2008). The interplay of on-going support of members and social activism within the greater community can imbue such alternatives with considerable distinctiveness.

The arts themselves are likely incorporated as a tool of activism rather than serving as a tool of therapy (Moxley et al., 2012). Alternative support structures can emerge from the arts, like the community arts studios. Such structures can foster creativity and activism among people who face considerable stigma. They can use the arts as a means of telling their stories, capturing the social forces that oppress them using image, voice, spoken word, lyrics, and dance. Studios may sponsor community exhibits the purpose of which is to communicate artists' perspectives to groups that can benefit from such enlightenment. Those group members may become secondary witnesses to the serious barriers, issues, and impediments faced by people who experience them routinely in their daily lives.

Those alternatives that incorporate the arts and humanities to advance an overarching critique of society and its human services may offer its members considerable leeway in structuring their critiques through the use of lyrics, visual portraitures, multimedia displays, and educational forums they connect with the arts. The use of narratives to tell alternative stories that challenge commonly accepted narratives may serve as a way of vocalizing what is not working for people, the consequences of stigma, and the truths behind marginalization. Arts-based alternatives may use innovative approaches to dissemination including exhibits to underscore inequities members experience. Artists themselves may interpret motifs for audiences, and can serve as docents of their own displays, or those of their peers. A principal idea driving such exhibits is presentation of art forms that educate audiences about the realities of the issues members must address in their daily lives.

Those systems or alternatives under professional control likely employ the arts as a tool of therapy, helping people express what they find problematic in their lives, and the consequences they experience as patients or clients. The arts become a tool of expression reinforcing the actual client labeling process in which a system produces unwanted consequences. Officials may implicate the misunderstanding of a given label by laypeople, those who do not understand the science of a particular disorder. The system itself likely refrains from implicating the issues the labeling process can create, something that is unlikely the focus of criticism professionals would engage in themselves, particularly in an age that legitimizes evidence under the control of professionals.

An Example of Degradation Within a Given Culture

Once I interacted with a young man who built a collage of the labeling process he experienced when a physician diagnosed him as Schizophrenic. Composing the collage were actual products that all held one thing in common: they degraded him personally, amplified his qualities they attributed to the diagnosis, and disparaged his identity if not his image as a young person striving for autonomy and self-definition. He laid each product on a timeline along butcher paper stretching almost 25 feet.

To form the collage, the young man included assessment reports, service plans, letters, and written professional opinions posting the artifacts to their appropriate dates. As I viewed the collage as a whole, I could see the multiple documents clumping at various ages. The clumps of documents emphasized limitations, deficits, and problems. Few if any spoke to the possibility for the young man achieving developmental milestones that are important at certain ages of the period society refers to as young adulthood. And few of the documents identified the young man's substantive strengths, which in his case involved imagination, creativity, creative expression and representation of ideas in visual form, and cultural criticism.

I felt a sickening sensation emerging in my gut as I walked along the considerable length of the collage, observing the various artifacts, and as I stepped back to see the collage as a whole. The official documents, the artifacts composing the collage, suggested collectively a principal arc: do not entertain any expectations since your disorder offers you little hope for the life you wanted for yourself before the onset of the labeling process itself.

The young man indicated to me that something was going on. That he had periods of what he called "real illness" challenging his functioning. But he did not see his situation as causing an abandonment of hope inherent in diminished expectations, and a life of illness.

This young man would likely be fine with a diagnosis of Schizophrenia if only it did not preclude life options he valued, and with which he was willing to struggle. Inherent in this story is a principal question I offer: What kind of culture could bestow a label for medication purposes, but leave open the life options inherent in the values and beliefs this young man possessed, and the social options that he valued, such as work, romantic attachment, relationships, education, and career?

This question, for me, is cultural, and the options I offer answer it in different ways. Adherents to the culture of *professional dominance* may argue that this young man's experience is indicative of poor quality in medical and psycho-social support. By improving the quality of care, the young man would benefit from qualified, astute, and skilled professionals who can change the arc of the young man's life course he communicated through the collage. Those who adhere to *enabling* would likely argue that the young man would benefit from representation that would resolve the issues he faces and achieve the kinds of support he wants for himself, or to be left alone and unharassed by professionals. The young man needs an effective representation that is not conflicted by the system seeking to help him, and is dedicated to the young man's interests as he defines them.

Alternatively, *the recipient-centered* adherent would argue for a team of competent professionals who can work closely with the young man to balance medical and psychosocial support. Members of the team would work together to empower the young man's voice, and they would listen closely to his strivings and desires. The medical professional would be one of several team members in which there are multiple perspectives helping this young man conceive of and implement a sound plan of community support balanced with his value of autonomy and his aim of independent living.

And then there is the *person-controlled* option. Here the overarching question for this young man is "Why do you want to stay in a system that neglects you, and abridges your desires for a full life." Adherents to this option would argue for an autonomous and independent consumer who may identify as a survivor of a system that marginalizes him. Assistance for these adherents would come in the form of a support system in which survivors work together to resist, oppose, and ignore a system that only seeks to limit their potential and autonomy.

Conclusion: Why is Consumerism Multi-Cultural in Human Services

The framework of cultural types offers some diversity in thinking about what constitutes a system of human services. Why does this diversity exist? My response is a political one. Given the nature of contemporary democracies, polities are struggling with the purpose and cost of human services. Open societies must be responsive to their citizens even though they may do so reluctantly given the considerable demands human services place on public resources. Consumerism suggests choice and options, and it underscores the collective focus of human services, as well as the necessity for respecting the autonomy and independence of consumers.

In the first chapter, I offer the values of voice and dissent as inherent in consumerism. Although these two values can conflict, as they often do in human services systems, professionals cannot easily harmonize them, although it is possible to do so within progressive approaches to consumer status and role. By diversifying cultures, human services as a societal institution can respect voice and dissent—they can allow for more empowered roles within human service systems, as well as offering would be consumers options to withdraw from established systems, actuate their own values, and find support in structures over which the systems themselves have little control.

Perhaps the limiting condition here is what the society offers through social welfare. Strong human and social rights frameworks in which there is considerable emphasis the society places on the adequacy of social provision (like housing, education, and income) can lower marginalization and allow people who would experience considerable marginalization to exercise their more idiographic qualities (i.e., those that do not adhere to normative standards or expectations). Their behavior would not influence their receipt of at least basic life resources.

Additionally, those societies that decriminalize certain behavioral forms, like illicit use of drugs, or sex work, and bring them into health care, or within a regulatory framework like public health, could reframe cultures of human services. Those cultures may engage in less social control, and seek to enhance the support of people who would want a range of social services or community support for themselves.

Of course, many societies are somewhat anxious about the policies of strong social rights, particularly those that detach work and social provision, like housing rents, as well as policies of decriminalization. Those societies likely shift the burden of human care and support from the general society (and its tax structures) to human service systems, making the response of those systems to social marginalization a significant challenge. Without ennobling social rights and the provisions flowing from them, the scope of human service systems will likely increase even in the face of Neoliberalism, and their social control features will be prominent. And this will result in diverse systems that are adjusting to the limited rights facing people who experience considerable marginalization.

References

Bockhoven, J. S. (1956). Moral treatment in American psychiatry. *Journal of Nervous and Mental Disease, 124*, 292–321.

Douglas, M., & Ney, S. (1998). *Missing person: A critique of personhood in the social sciences*. Russel Sage Foundation.

Moxley, D., & Freddolino, P. (1990, September). A model of advocacy for promoting client self-determination in psychosocial rehabilitation. *Psychosocial Rehabilitation Journal, 14*(2), 69–82.

Moxley, D., & Freddolino, P. (1994, June). Client-driven advocacy and psychiatric disability: A Model for social work practice. *Journal of Sociology and Social Welfare, 21*(2), 98–108.

Moxley, D., & Paul, M. (2005, May). Advocacy and guardianship. In W. Crimando & T. F. Riggar (Eds.), *Community resources: A practical guide for human service professionals* (pp. 200–217). Waveland Press.

Moxley, D. P., Feen-Calligan, H., & Washington, O. G. M. (2012, July). Lessons learned from three projects linking social work, the arts and humanities. *Social Work Education: the International Journal, 31*(6), 703–723.

Stern, G. (2012). School superintendents call for tougher gun control, mental health funding. *Lohud.com*. Retrieved December 20, 2012, from http://www.lohud.com/article/20121231/NEWS/312310066/School-superintendents-call-tougher-gun-control-mental-health-funding

Teplin, L., McClelland, G., Abram, K., & Weiner, D. (2005). Crime victimization in adults with severe mental illness: Comparison with the National Crime Victimization Survey. *Archives of General Psychiatry, 62*, 911–921.

Viebeck, E. (2012, December 21). Catholic bishops call for gun control, mental health reforms. *Healthwatch*. Retrieved December 24, 2012, from http://thehill.com/blogs/healthwatch/mental-health/274235-catholic-bishops-call-for-gun-control-mental-health-reform

Washington, O., & Moxley, D. (2008). Telling my story: From narrative to exhibit in illuminating the lived experience of homelessness among older African American women. *Journal of Health Psychology, 13*(2), 154–165.

6

The Inside-Outside Approach to Consumerism

Introduction

While the person-driven culture may exist within established human service systems (such as in the case of medication-free treatment programs in mental health care), they more likely exist outside of the confines of human service systems and are voluntarily created by their members who find refuge in a group life they control. This culture and the corresponding alternative (the enabling one) I identify in Fig. 4.1 (Quadrants I and II) very likely represent what I call the outside pole of the inside-outside dimension of consumerism. They likely exist outside of human service systems because their members seek a radical alternative to prevailing norms and requirements those systems may stipulate. Established human service professionals may dismiss such alternatives as aberrations since they nullify dominant conceptions of how best to respond to human needs.

The existence of alternatives outside of formal human service systems reminds us that most human service systems do not fully incorporate nor address all of the social forces involved in producing human need. For some (those who affiliate with human service systems) likely attribute some measure of legitimacy to those systems while for others, those who disaffiliate from such systems, and may delegitimize them, view the outsider position quite essential to activism. For it is the outside that we can witness the operation of dissent in the support systems and advocacy options those entities can produce on behalf of their members.

That those outside options are not driven by professional necessity as their criterion for offering support, enabling and person-driven cultures may offer a broader array of support that may more readily address the negative social consequences people living with the label of illness, disability or deviance may experience within established systems. Consumerism in the physical health domain (e.g., in cardiac illness, diabetes, pulmonary health, and arthritis) also reveals the importance of addressing the negative social consequences that illness can create, thereby revealing the shortcomings of human services steeped in the medical model. Health is much broader than medical status alone. In general, avenues of social support, stress reduction, enhanced social services, and access to income and modified employment reflect important ways for facilitating healing. Perhaps it is best to view health as situations in which people can fulfill their daily living needs in ways that bring about quality of day, based on either normative considerations or those idiographic ones fulfilling the aims individuals establish for themselves.

Reducing the number and severity of issues people experience as a result of their status may result in a net reduction of stress. The alleviation of distress—or better yet the prevention of or early resolution of those issues producing distress—may be one of the best principal strategies for producing positive health outcomes inherent in well-being and flourishing. Identifying and resolving as early as possible impediments to good housing, desired employment and education, and ongoing social support may be sound remedies for the issues many people with diminished status face in their daily lives. And, by placing those responses under the direct control of people who experience them, equipping them with options to sustain their own organizational structures (such as through the use of community block grant dollars, local public human service funds, local tax revenue, or even vouchers), the cultures of enabling or person-driven support may truly bring about the kind of empowerment many human service professions often assert as important.

Those options that cluster around the outsider perspective may be as much a part of policy as those options that constitute the insider perspective. Policies may address the extent to which entities outside of formal human services can evolve. And while policies enfranchise the development of formal systems, they may also respect alternatives that bring other options into existence outside of those systems.

Consumerism Within Human Service Organizations and Systems

When one considers the insider view of consumerism, what is striking is the expansion of roles available to recipients, although there is some question about the institutionalization of such roles within those systems. My own research indicates that people who are brought into formal support roles, like case aides or peer support specialists, or in formal treatment roles, like prosumers (those who combine roles as consumers who have completed formal education in a human service discipline) may face numerous cultural, attitudinal, or credentialing barriers to establishing themselves as bona fide providers of peer support. My colleague, Dr. Carol Mowbray, and I along with several colleagues examined the expansion of mental health support systems for people coping with severe and persistent mental illness through the incorporation of people who were in recovery as vocational support specialists. Those specialists offered assistance to recipients in job search strategies, sustaining a job search, and securing a job.

The recipients themselves wanted to pursue employment and to modify those employment opportunities to offer them some flexibility in light of the personal issues they experienced as a result of their illness. Introducing those new roles into established programs in which professionals serve in core staffing positions reflects the kind of consumerism consistent with an internal approach. In this case, the sponsoring organizations were seeking to be responsive to the employment aims of those recipients who were in recovery. Thus, the idea of role expansion is indicative of this kind of approach to consumerism.

There are other ways a human service system can go about its approach to consumerism. For example, it could have established a program or organization operated for and by consumers who would support the vocational development, work experience, and employment of people who have moved through a formal process of professional treatment. The professional staff within an organization could make internal referrals to that program mindful that those they refer would meet certain criteria of appropriateness. The programmatic or organizational alternative remains under professional and organizational control incorporating criteria of diagnostic appropriateness, progress in recovery, and readiness as decision tools in moving people forward toward employment.

One can observe the same dynamics in those entities offering "person first" options such as housing first. In this programmatic alternative, people who are homeless obtain housing first by virtue of their need without the obligation on their part of demonstrating their sincerity or their willingness to participate in professional treatment. Personnel practicing such a philosophy are willing to offer support to residents to hold on to their housing, and to promote continuity of the placement. The professional staff may practice a person-centered or recipient-centered kind of approach to the provision of support. The staff members are likely very interested in what a person wants to achieve for themselves, and may offer considerable social support in helping the person achieve goals that they find meaningful.

Consumerism within a human service system reflects certain core values that are consistent with a progressive orientation to the provision of care, treatment, and support. *Humanism* is dominant within the internal approach in which there is considerable concern for what a person wants for themselves and how those aspirations are tied to their culture, ethnicity, gender, class, or sexuality. Professional interest is invested in discerning those desires on part of the people professional staff serve or otherwise support. In this approach, professionals are consultative. They bring their specialized professional knowledge to bear in helping people make decisions that are in their *best interests*. It is the focus on best interests in which professionals help people balance risk and success in making informed choices about what they want to achieve through their own efforts and professional support. Consumerism in this way preserves the power and sanctity of professional power or influence. Both humanism and a best interests approach form the basis of *respect* professionals offer the people whom they assist.

In this sense the internal approach to consumerism is conciliatory. It seeks to help consumers through nonconflictual means in which professionals see the needs of people who are enrolled in human service as ones they are willing to address, and ones that are possible as long as the recipients are reasonable actors within the established system—that is, they do not ask for more than the system can deliver. In other words, consumerism works when people in need, that is, recipients, play the established game in which professionals in helping roles remain in control of the system in which the game unfolds. The ritualism that often operates in such systems is part of the system's culture and preserves the collaborative equilibrium of the system. The internal consumer culture embodies humanism, best interests, and respect that form the game of collaborative exchange between professionals and recipients.

When I refer to a client- or recipient-centered approach, I am suggesting that the desires or wishes of those in care do not necessarily drive the system culture. Certainly, needs either broadly or narrowly construed by professionals do serve as advanced organizers of care. Other considerations, however, may be more potent in established service cultures, like medical necessity in which recipients or potential recipients must meet or surpass a professionally defined threshold of severity of need. For some individuals, like in certain housing programs, if a person will not likely qualify for the receipt of housing, if they fail to achieve certain diagnostic criteria and the thresholds of functioning that go along with an appropriate diagnosis, then they are ineligible. Diagnostic differentiation may determine medical necessity (as opposed to social necessity).

Alternatively, an internal approach to consumerism may incorporate values that form a tension with diagnostic differentiation like policies involving a philosophy of "no wrong door," wrap around, and "zero reject." No wrong door means that whomever enters a human service organization will receive a modicum of support even though they may not fit the diagnostic profile established by the organization. More generalist-oriented human service organizations, especially ones serving particular communities, and in this sense are locality-based, and locality-focused, may receive anyone who comes to the doors of those organizations in search of assistance.

People who face numerous complex issues, who lack support, and who are mired in very challenging life situations, like poverty, may receive wraparound support from such entities. These organizations offer cultures in which comprehensive social, health, and rehabilitative services can be mustered to address complex human problems brought to those organizations by individuals who experience considerable vulnerability. Ultimately, these organizations may incorporate an overarching policy best referred to as "zero reject." They relax if not eliminate rigid eligibility criteria, assess needs and situations quickly, employ staff members who appear very much like recipients in race, demeanor, clothing, and language, and have facilities that one could call street level—that is, they are easily accessible in location, and likely their appearance does not escalate someone's anxiety.

Such locality-based organizations are likely a good reflection of an internal approach to consumerism. Their comprehensive approach to accessibility is one of their strengths, and people in need likely feel safe in approaching them for assistance and becoming a recipient within them. One can argue that rather than professional control operating as a core strategy in such organizations, an approach to locality-based responsiveness is more operative.

There is an inherent tension between professional dominance and recipient-centered approaches to internal consumerism. Tempering professional dominance can be new kinds of recipient roles and new kinds of rituals that place the recipient at the center of care even though challenging this can be greater organizational efforts to offer support in efficient ways that remain under the ultimate control of professionals. Such an organization will probably struggle with tensions forming between professionals who see themselves as possessing the knowledge and skill in responding to human needs in particular ways and recipients who want to have greater say (i.e., voice) in how they are treated and in what they receive. This tension can be a good one in that it illuminates the dynamics of relationships between professionals and consumers. The tension, however, can produce conflict requiring productive organizational responses.

The locality-based organization is concerned about being present within a given locale and responding to the needs of the locale as a whole. Perhaps a central idea in locality based organizations is attributed need—if the community as a whole experiences elevated negative social indicators, then helpers assume that those who reside in that community possess heightened risk for bad life outcomes. Criticism may be directed to such an organization because of its flexibility and fluidity. Critics may argue that the organization is deprofessionalized, and does not possess the expertise to address the depth of human need existing within a particular community. This may be true. Such organizations may lack high levels of professional staffing with an absence of specialized knowledge from education, training, and credentialing. But what the organization loses in professional capacity it may gain in sensitivity, responsiveness, and innovation in addressing those needs manifest within households, families, groups, and individuals that are heightened because of the marginalization of the community the organization serves.

One may observe two mechanisms at work when consumerism occurs within human service organizations and systems. First, there can be complementarity in which role expansion and innovation on the part of recipients complements the work of highly credentialed professionals. *Complementarity* means that what recipients as helpers can offer complements already established protocol for professional helping. Complementarity does not mean that recipients as helpers are primary, indeed, they are likely secondary. They assist professionals in responding to the needs of consumers. At best, recipients are assistants.

Second, there can be *extension*. Recipients as helpers extend the system of support compensating for the limitations in time and flexibility of professional staff. Extension can manifest in extending the availability of support across time, day, and weeks. Such extension may create new kinds of supportive environments or situations like drop-in centers, warm lines, and outreach to households or the streets. Complementarity and extension are what I call progressive since they reduce the social distance between the organization and its professional staff and recipients, can make the system more responsive and sensitive to the issues recipients bring, and likely expand the roles of recipients within the process of care, treatment, and support.

Consumerism Outside of Human Service Organizations and Systems

My previous discussion of the insider approach to consumerism legitimizes professionals. For the most part, consumerism outside of human service organizations and systems delegitimize human service professionals. They reduce the influence of professionals if not vitiate them as irrelevant or even as dangerous. One argument I have stated before is that the professions within health and human services, particularly those addressing the needs of people who are emotionally, cognitively, experientially, or behaviorally different, serve almost exclusively social control purposes.

In this sense, societal agents see people who are different as potential or real threats to the greater society, and must be dealt with in ways to contain their threat. If a person's appearance or conduct or modes of interacting appear grossly different from the norm, then the community must address such deviance. Doing so may implicate humanistic approaches such as diverting people to humane treatment within human service systems. Or doing so may be draconian involving incarceration or isolation. Indeed, isolation or expulsion may be one of the cruelest forms of control since it can remove people from environments that can stimulate their senses, decrease deprivation that compromises health, and foster their further development.

Consumerism has formed in such a crucible involving marginalization, oppression, or wholesale rejection of people having certain qualities, like cognitive ones that the greater society views as odd or even extreme. Consumerism in this vein can result in the founding of innovative support systems or even formal organizations that embody counter-cultural values, affirm those who are disaffirmed within public spaces, and who may be harmed by the enforcement of rules and laws to coerce their behavior or remove them from public visibility.

What may emerge from such innovation is considerable creativity and creative community building, particularly within a framework of mutual support or self-help. Mutual support can augment those resources the greater society may eliminate or retrench. First, mutual support can offer avenues for affirmation amplifying people's personal qualities as important sources of self-concept and self-esteem. By doing so, mutual support can replace isolation with sociability offering people sanctuary or refuge from a world in which they are unwanted. Mutual support can help augment information, help people gain insight into the issues and the negative consequences society creates for those who must shoulder those issues, and create group cohesion through a shared grand narrative about how society disenfranchises people who come to know themselves as unwanted. It is in reframing the sense of personal agency that mutual support may serve as a powerful source of transformation. Indeed, we may refer to the resulting personal agency as empowerment.

Salient within the outsider form of consumerism is the absence of professionals or the marginalization of professionals. They are not seen as a source of solutions, but rather as the source of the problems they create for people whose perceived or real differences set them apart from the mainstream. The outsider form may eschew the mainstream and therefore there is a rejection of professionals because of their complicity in enforcing mainstream norms. Oftentimes, the stories of outsiders are replete with condemnation of the normative roles of professionals in sustaining the status quo, as opposed to professionals promoting and respecting diversity in cognition, behavior, emotion, and lifestyles as an expression of a multi-cultural society. In this sense, the outsider form of consumerism manifests in support groups and the organizations that embody them serve as a defense against normativity. They also can be a defense against criminalization of those who are deprived or oppressed. The wholesale rejection of certain groups, especially manifest in geographic segregation, isolation, and the deprivation of material sustenance, can ensue.

Self-help extends from mutual support since cohesion among groups likely generates social action. It can equip those who face discrimination and its accompanying deprivation with skills and competencies to take action on their own or in concert with groups. Here social action may be a potent form of self-help involving the development of activists, and the empowerment of their assertiveness to confront injustices at local and governmental levels. The confrontation of injustice, particularly its institutionalization, may be the ultimate expression of this form of consumerism.

Self-help leans on the empowerment of those who engage in it. The expression of empowerment demands psychological, group, and organizational capacities. At a psychological level, people call upon virtues like courage and tenacity. And, self-efficacy, an internalized belief that one can bring about the outcomes they desire, can figure into the process of action. The embodiment of these psychological capacities within groups can strengthen resolve, follow-through, and action. Mutual support can serve as a sustaining factor in mobilizing social action the purpose of which is likely institutional: those on the outside may confront institutional representatives to change, or at least produce embarrassment or shame in how they treat the so-called other.

Born from social action, public awareness building, and the condemnation of public officials, organizations can form from these social movements that compete with established human service organizations. Not only may these organizations introduce a new critical narrative about social issues experienced by those who engage in dissent, but also they can offer alternative programs of action, especially ones that promote novel pathways to addressing the social issues once under the exclusive control of professionals and their organizations. These organizations likely offer alternative cultures and alternative support systems.

At least two different strategies are operative in the outside form of consumerism. The first and oftentimes the most salient is the formation of mutual support groups and systems among people who face marginalization. These mutual support groups may be discrete bringing people together in libraries, restaurants, or churches to discuss commonalities in experience and situations. People may open their homes to members of the groups. Some support groups may remain private since public scrutiny could jeopardize employment, livelihoods, education, and professional standing. Public scrutiny could literally destroy a person's reputation.

Alternatively, mutual support may be quite public and, in addition to supporting its members individually and collectively, groups may push out their program into the public sphere through the arts and performance. Some mutual support groups can coalesce into whole communities in which members share shelter, food, recreation, and cultural enrichment. The advent of homeless camps, urban farms, and businesses indicates that mutual support can occur at higher levels of organizational development for certain groups. Witness the business movement among Deaf and Deafened individuals as a sound example of such organization. Businesses can serve more as social enterprises rather than exclusively money-making schemes. Social enterprises can blend community service, business activity, and mutual support offering innovations in social relations and community development.

The second strategy is social activism. Mutual support can evolve quickly into social protest and even more intrusive forms of activism, like boycotts and public criticism of corporations, institutions, like churches or universities, and politicians. Mutual support can build bonds among members and strengthen trust. Events outside of the group can catalyze action directing the energy of the members into confrontation and protest. Chaining themselves to buses to protest the absence of accessible transportation, people who have physical disabilities, and who are dependent on public transportation, can disrupt urban infrastructure, and make their point salient in the media and to observing members of the public. The police force that intercedes and is seen dragging people from the scene of protest makes the point for the protesting group. The advent of social media may underscore with immediacy such actions, and bring into question how communities are responding to people who experience inequities and injustice.

Social protest as disruption is a potent form of engagement in the outsider form of consumerism. Action can frustrate public decision-makers, challenge law enforcement, embarrass officials, and reveal the social order of discrimination. Although protest can potentially result in the arrest and confinement of activists, a well-organized protest anticipates this eventuality. Arrest and subsequent arraignment or incarceration become part of the protest, and perhaps a powerful part. Here again social media and other forms of media can communicate vividly the sources of injustice particular groups face. A special form of media attention is particularly potent: the use of media for the purposes of expose. Documentary, news coverage that turns into a series, and the amplification of injustice by print media can increase public awareness and move public officials to action. Protest can make visible what many people within the mainstream may wish to ignore or suppress. Activists understand public deniability and seek to fix public responsibility for the purposes of social change that favors their group.

So, the outsider form of consumerism is by most measures not conciliatory. Those who are outsiders do not seek rapprochement with human service professionals. The two expressions of the outsider form involve *withdraw* and/or *confrontation*. In the former, outsiders found their own support systems and develop their own organizations. Mutual support that builds a strong membership is operative here. Like any form of group life, mutual support can produce cohesion, a solidarity among members that they are not the problem in society, but rather society produces problems for members. In the latter, confrontation is a powerful form not only of public self-expression but also of assertive demands for change. The commonality connecting these two expressions of the outsider form is the delegitimization of professionals. They simply are not primary to the experience of those who are marginalized. Rather than valorizing professionals, it is best to promote the interests and competencies of those who have been marginalized.

Two mechanisms may operate when consumerism occurs outside of human service systems, when it is undertaken by those who consider themselves survivors, or victims of prejudice or discrimination in the greater society. One is *enhancement* involving the elevation of the status of the people who are labeled as problematic or dependent. Enhancement can come about through legal action, social action, and accompanying policy change. A second is *substitution* when the outsiders found their own entities to promote their well-being irrespective of what a professional class seeks through human services. Substitution creates an alternative pathway through society in the provision of mutual support and the realization of self-help.

Conclusion: Ins and Outs of Consumerism and Survivorship

I consider the mechanisms of complementarity and extension to be progressive ones since they fall within the internal expression of consumerism. These two mechanisms can advance the humanism of a human service system, soften the rigidity of formal organizations, particularly bureaucracies, and enhance the voice of those who obtain assistance. Alternatively, I consider the mechanisms of enhancement and substitution to serve as radicalization of social welfare policy since they restructure the power between those who experience marginalization and those in power who either bring marginalization about or influence its presence within society.

All four mechanisms offer policy alternatives within human services. The mechanisms can promote systems change within human service organizations or create alternatives to professionally controlled systems of care, treatment, and support. I consider these mechanisms within the context of a policy framework I offer in the next chapter.

7

Progressive and Radical Policy Strategies

Introduction

Earlier in this monograph, I offer the question of "What constitutes a contemporary human service system defined principally by its adherents and its dissidents?" The typology I offer differentiates between *adherents*, those recipients who endorse the system, and those survivors or *dissidents* who remove themselves from such systems either to exert influence over their reform, to live their lives without what they see as official interference, or move on to found support systems in which survivors adopt counter-official narratives. Within this typology I differentiate between the establishment and expression of statuses and related roles I identify as consumer recipients and survivors.

The four cultures I offer in a previous chapter hold implications for social welfare policy, and strategies communities could use to legitimize consumerism within established systems of human services, or pathways offering people alternatives as consumers. Such a differential framework moves one from programmatic and organizational considerations to policy ones. Here I consider policy as those frameworks in which a particular society defines its relationship (either positive or negative) with those

© The Author(s), under exclusive license to Springer Nature Singapore Pte Ltd. 2021
D. P. Moxley, *Consumerism in the Human Services*,
https://doi.org/10.1007/978-981-16-7192-0_7

individuals who are members of the society, citizens, or those who do not have formal standing. This relationship may be highly structured in the sense of the provision of benefits to those members, the definition of statuses in which all people or certain groups can expect particular benefits, and people who could expect certain institutional responses, whether those are negative or positive.

Social welfare policy can recognize human needs at various levels whether survival-oriented ones, requiring immediate or even crisis responses, supportive requirements for people who may be unable to participate in job markets, or those that require certain kinds of social supports because of their status of dependency, or developmental ones that help people address their aspirations, typically through the enhancement of opportunity structures, like education. This considerable variation in social welfare policy suggests that societies possess different approaches to meeting human needs. This variation likely extends from the overarching culture of a society that defines the relationship between individuals, groups, and communities and the greater society.

The cultures structuring the relationships between consumer recipients and human service systems are an expression of social welfare policy as is the cultures structuring relationships between survivors and human service systems. That structuring expresses itself as a spectrum of statuses and related roles potentially adding considerable diversity to the scope of social welfare policy. This diversity has certain advantages. It offers roles and opportunity structures (perhaps novel ones) for those individuals who remain within existing systems of human services, and who seek to expand their own involvement in how those systems operate, and in how they relate to other recipients of support, benefits, and opportunities. The value of empowerment can influence the structuring of those statuses and roles and how those roles create opportunities for individuals who enact them in their daily lives as consumer recipients or even as survivors whose claims are built into prevailing social welfare institutions.

The cultures structuring the relationships between survivors and human service systems are more ambiguous. I say this because survivors may adopt two action frames. For survivors one frame may define their relationships with providers of human services as an *adversarial* one in which survivors generate considerable conflict, raising issues about the legitimacy of human services, in terms of both the means of provision and the outcomes they seek to bring about. A second frame involves survivors who *withdraw* from any voluntary or societally enforced consumption or use of human services. As I have noted in previous chapters, this frame legitimizes the founding of potentially alternative support systems.

Human Management Models as Derivative of Social Welfare Policy

Whether people seek opportunities through human services or seek to reject prevailing options of human services implicate peoples' responses to human management. Some may disagree with me here, but social welfare policies produce human management options. For a society, human dependency amplifies certain value orientations a society applies in responding to human need. Those human management models may be very controlling seeking to confine people within certain areas of a community, or within institutions or organizations. This confinement is a cultural response with derivative implications for the scope of social institutions, and following from such responses can be particular human management models. The models themselves facilitate or otherwise enable societal aims. Social welfare policy is an expression of those aims, and can produce human management models to achieve those aims.

Videographer Frederick Wiseman illuminates the contours of those human service models through his documentary work (Grant, 2006). These are worth viewing since his videography reveals how human management models work in the daily lives of the people who are immersed in them, including those who are the recipients and those who serve either in helping roles or in supervisory roles, like detention officers. *Titicut Follies* (Wiseman, 1967) is one of the most provocative of Wiseman's videographies. It shows graphically the operations of a forensic psychiatric facility and reveals in detail, oftentimes gruesome detail, the relationships between inmates and those who supervise them.

The videographic detail reveals the paradigmatic form of facility and degradation as a standing feature involving rigid routines of daily life, and their degradation, and the abuse, neglect, and deprivation the inmates' routine experience. I use this example to suggest that human management models do not necessarily express themselves in positive ways. Indeed, human management models may serve the purposes of removing people from the mainstream of society, isolating them, and depriving them of decent or dignified care or treatment.

Wiseman's other videos illuminate the operations of yet other human management models in American society. *Public Housing* (Wiseman, 1997) captures the cacophony of a public housing site in an American city. The relationships between police officers and residents, the patrolling of the housing site, and the adjacent community reveal the considerable stress operating within the area for residents, community members, and police officers. Wiseman captures a given situation visually through the use of video, and he yields to viewers the responsibility for interpretation. For me, this documentary is a glaring example of segregation in which a particular group, a minority within American society, experiences intentional management by the greater society, one enforced by social welfare policy, and one in which social welfare policy interacts with policing and law enforcement. Segregation of certain groups has been for a long time central to the aims of social policy in the United States.

There are two other human management models Wiseman reveals in his videography. In *Adjustment and Work* (Wiseman, 1986), the videographer reveals the operations of a technical facility whose participants possess sensory differences, the facility personnel, members of educational institutions, and American social welfare policy would call impairments. The video illuminates the various processes professionals use to help people "adjust to their impairments," and "adjust" to American society. The routines incorporate personal assessment, vocational evaluation, career preparation, and employment and training. The portrayal reminds me how adjustment is central to social welfare as an aim. This distinctive human management model focuses on how people must compensate for their impairment with the aim of either engagement in productive activity, and/or participation in American society.

Wiseman offers videographic studies that for me reveal yet other human management models. These include *High School I* (1968), *High School II* (1994), and *Welfare* (1975). The models remind viewers that

American society, and actually all societies, structures their relationships with those individuals who are "impaired" and therefore design and implement specialized environments so their impairment does not disrupt the routines of the greater community.

Wolfensberger articulated archetypal forms influencing societal responses to impairment and dependency. What he calls institutional models—and those I refer to as human management models—can embody particular value systems (and visible in their architecture, routines, rituals, and staffing). To paraphrase Wolfensberger, those archetypes involve infantilization of the recipient, the framing of recipient as angelic, or the framing of recipient as dangerous. Later when Wolfensberger introduced his framework of social role valorization he offered another archetype—the so-called impaired person as a competent human being. This idea of competence is central to a consideration of consumerism as a way of correcting for the overreaching control of individuals and groups by society (through policy) and its social institutions.

Competent individuals should have considerable control over their lives, chart their own path toward an end they wish, receive support they want to activate their path, and achieve their ends. These aims are central to what many human service professions refer to as self-determination. Whether individuals want professional involvement, peer support, or live by their own devices is best left up to individuals, even though there is always the possibility of societal intervention. Often such intervention (or intrusion) is legally mediated, when societal agents determine that people cannot care for themselves, are dangerous, or engage in conduct or behavior that is found revolting to others.

The latter occurs when society stipulates a strict physical bodily form that flows from a given aesthetic. Deviation from such aesthetic can be seen by others as problematic and a cause for the exertion of social control, oftentimes through enforced isolation or removal from mainstream community life. From the standpoint of a broader conception of consumerism within society, this determination should not be the central nor the principal way of structuring the relationship between people in need and the greater society. The response should be residual. It should follow from the exhaustion of supportive alternatives that are under the control of individuals who are otherwise seen as impaired, unwanted, or useless by the greater society and its agents.

The value orientation of the greater society and its translation (through legislation, code, regulations, and other rule systems) of this orientation into social welfare policy and related human management models can shape that society's conception of consumerism. I argue that consumerism broadly conceived in health and human service systems is in response to human management models that are too restrictive, pursue nefarious aims, limit the freedom of individuals, and devolve into forms of human neglect and abuse.

A policy of consumerism introduces diverse human management models. Within human service systems, those models broaden participation of recipients, promote co-production among all actors, and restructure the relationships between recipients and professionals. Outside of human services systems, those models broaden control of would-be recipients over their own support systems likely resulting in the elimination of the influence of human service professionals, demedicalization of the problems of daily living, and the creation of narratives under control of survivors or those who eschew public involvement in their daily lives. Videographic documentation of those human management models could reveal properties and qualities very different from those Wiseman offers in his tremendously powerful documentaries of existing societal arrangements for people society considers dangerous, impaired, useless, or unwanted.

Positive Human Management Models

There is the possibility of creating positive human management models in the face of despair. "After Goodbye: An AIDS Story," produced by KERA, a nonprofit media organization in Texas, documents the considerable loss of the members of the Turtle Creek Chorale because of AIDS. The chorale itself offers members a source of creative engagement and the group support accompanying it. Not only does the video address death and dying of members due to AIDS, and their impact on the surviving members, it examines Gay culture at a group level, and how members use the performing arts to build support among them.

"After Goodbye" is an exemplar of mutual support under the control of members, forming naturally from mutual interests among the members in music and song. The video features "When we no longer touch" that examines the grieving process among members, and reveals their resilience and considerable fortitude. Such virtues draw members together and form a cohesion that itself is a healing factor when people face existential threat.

Why do I conceive of this exemplar as a human management model? In the previous chapter, I shared ones that are quite negative. They control members, enforce segregation, strip amenities from daily life, and diminish the quality of environment. Alternatively, the chorale exerts group support and a positive aesthetic in the face of threat. Gay men join together in a self-protective fashion and build resilience even in the face of death. Some 90 members succumbed to death by complications AIDS brought about.

The positive aesthetic distinguishes this kind of human management model from negative ones. A positive model is likely membership-based—people come together voluntarily to manage not only a threat but also the consequences of that threat. Or, the members join together to address the stigma they experience in the outside world. Those viewing "After Goodbye" will observe the edgy humor among the members who must deal with the health-compromising effects of AIDS, but who must also face discrimination and stigma at the hands of family members, relatives, and neighbors. Metaphorically, the positive aesthetic is a wall of sorts the members erect to protect and manage themselves in the face of both physiological and social threats.

Animating the chorale, one may argue, is not only AIDS but also the social reaction members experience as Gay men. Even in a stigma-free world, and one free of AIDS, one would likely find a group whose members are Gay. They would likely come together for the purposes of supporting their shared interests, and their common identity. The formation of such communities is an expression of pluralism. Diverse groups can find their own paths toward self-fulfillment, and even flourish in the face of societal rejection and neglect.

What are the indicants of a positive human management model? I offer the following:

1. Evident in the structure is a membership of people who come together to share mutual support.
2. A positive aesthetic forms to counter the negative aesthetic the greater society exerts.
3. The culture reinforces a common positive identity among members.
4. Cohesion is strong reinforcing the ties of mutual support and affinity among members.
5. There is a program that unites members into a positive group life.
6. Members are willing to advocate for a cause they find essential to their well-being.
7. The positive aesthetic contributes to a positive and fulfilling quality of day and quality of life.

Progressive and Radical Policy Alternatives in Fostering Consumerism

Potential strategies social welfare policy can embrace can produce considerable real or potential heterogeneity depending on which ones a particular system emphasizes or blends together as a result of its value base. Taking the empowerment of either consumers or survivors (or both) statuses as a principal overarching aim of that policy to ensure multiple avenues through which people can achieve their own preferences for support and realize outcomes they value, the policy itself can come to realize *progressive values* (ones that seek to humanize health and human service systems through an elaboration of consumer support or participation that affirm system and organizational goals) or *radical values* (ones that foster dissent, critical consciousness, and alternative opportunity structures under the control of members). The establishment of those strategies may express themselves within or outside of existing systems through two progressive options and two radical alternatives I offer in Table 7.1. The table captures the policy options I offer in this chapter.

Table 7.1 Progressive and radical strategies

Strategy	Policy aims and rationale	Organizational forms	Statuses and roles of participants
Progressive options: *Consumer recipient* *alternatives*			
Complementarity	These alternatives offer an opportunity structure for people with experiencing the causes and consequences of social issues to humanize care through incorporation of considerable role innovation.	These alternatives operate within human service systems and are nested within existing organizations and programs. So, for example, consumers may be involved in offering on-going support within case management programs, Assertive Community Treatment teams, vocational development opportunities, and housing options.	The consumer fills a quasi-helping role likely with considerable ambiguity attached to the status and role. The consumer may adopt a title like "prosumer" in which incumbents see themselves as integrating professional responsibilities with the insights they have gained from their first-person experience with the system. Here the Peer Support Specialist or Peer Support Recovery Specialist may be prominent.
Extension	These alternatives offer alternative opportunity structures for consumer recipients. Their aim is to humanize the system by offering environments that extend support beyond what people receive within established medical programs like medication clinics and case management. The option humanizes the system by addressing what professionals define as problematic consequences of degraded status like the experience of isolation, diminished social networks, and loss of motivation for social involvement. Professionals may treat those social states as persistent symptoms of a person's problem in daily living.	Human service systems can foster organizational development that extends support for consumer recipients outside of existing core programs. These options may be within or outside of the system but nonetheless their intent is to confine involvement to people with appropriate diagnostic statuses in extended social support opportunities under the control of professional staff. Examples include consumer-operated drop-in centers and clubhouses.	The consumer recipient stands as a member of an entity that facilitates involvement in options that augment social support, involvement, and integration as well as role performance. Participants have visible roles in the governance and operation of programmatic options and their helping efforts emanate from their roles as members. Self-help emerges from membership.

(continued)

Table 7.1 continued

Strategy	Policy aims and rationale	Organizational forms	Statuses and roles of participants
Radical options: Ex-patient or survivor alternatives			
Enhancement	Such alternatives enhance the status and role of the person who possesses a degraded label or even identity. They go beyond the offer of an opportunity structure to an advocacy option that helps individuals address the serious and high magnitude issues they face typically as a result of carrying the degraded label. Thus, the alternative here addresses issues that result from discrimination and oppression. The idea is that as a result of the labeling process people experience numerous intractable issues (e.g., housing or employment discrimination) they cannot resolve alone.	Typically operating outside of existing systems, these options may be organized as entities that offer (1) legal alternatives, (2) lay or professional advocacy, or (3) enhanced representation. They may incorporate enabling cultures in which professionals may act on behalf of the individual who specifies the result or outcomes they seek. Or, they may incorporate person-driven cultures in which the organization prepares people to take action on their own behalf with considerable control over the kinds of support they receive to enact empowered action.	This strategy incorporates a conception of status in which the person is a client almost in a legal sense. The helper is devoted solely to that which the person seeks to achieve and the helper operates without conflicting loyalties inherent in the roles of professionals who deliver care through human service system. As a client, the person exercises control over the direction of the advocacy or action, and specifies to the helper what is desired. Participants may conceive of themselves as survivors of the system and their treatment as well as the serious issues they face. Enhancement seeks to empower the status of the person by focusing on their (1) framing of the issues they face, (2) identification of the outcomes they seek, and (3) an enhancement of the control they exercise over the helping process and its goals.

(continued)

Table 7.1 continued

Strategy	Policy aims and rationale	Organizational forms	Statuses and roles of participants
Substitution	That this strategic option substitutes survivor-operated support systems for existing human service programs and arrangements makes it distinctive within social welfare policy. Substitution incorporates a critique of the existing system and its policies and practices. It likely embodies a grand narrative concerning discrimination, oppression, and marginalization emanating out of social control. The option stands in opposition to established systems offering participants opportunities for mobilization, dissent, campaigns, and social action.	Organizational forms can be quite diverse. Diversity is manifest in on-going social support systems extending into the operation of housing opportunities, employment, and social activism, which is one way an organization operationalizes dissent. Cultural development through the incorporation of performance, arts, and critical discourse can further strengthen identity. Identity formation (e.g., participants as survivors) may be an important cultural effect sought by such entities.	Participants can emerge as empowered actors within this option who find the identity as survivors quite fitting as a way of affirming their realities and self-conceptions. Holding statuses as empowered actors who command considerable influence within their settings is an outcome of the leadership, involvement, and enculturation they realize within the organizations with which they affiliate. A participant may have a diverse role set involving provider and recipient of support, administrator, fund developer, and/or governor. And, they may gain statuses and roles as outcomes of the support they receive—such as worker, tenant, and student.

Progressive Policy Strategies

Progressive strategies (involving *complementarity* and *extension*) seek to humanize an existing system by helping recipients interact with one another as sources of support and address what health and human service providers conceive as enduring negative symptoms of the issues that bring them into a system of care. Taken together, the two policy strategies affirm that consumerism can extend what human service providers offer their recipients, and complement the roles of professionals with minimal if no disruption. Consumerism in this sense adds value to professional roles and can increase coverage of groups, increase social productivity within existing systems, and foster alternative cultures of social interaction. Here humanization can embrace the expansion of role options for recipients involving membership, mutual support, and peer helping activities achieved through the integration of peer support roles within established human services.

Such expansion actually complements helping activities undertaken by professionals. Consumerism does not threaten the status of professionals and can, in fact, strengthen their status since the system may not honor the helping arrangements flowing from consumerism as central to the well-being of recipients. The systems may see those arrangements as expression of folk culture, healing options emerging from various group identities, like indigenous sources, as adjunctive, as peripheral, or worse, as lacking relevance. That those options may occur during times and periods of the week in which professionals are unavailable may make them peripheral.

The progressive human service professional in such contexts endorses and facilitates such role expansion and may herald a system that is more balanced reflecting a differentiation in helping allocated among peers and professionals. However, such role innovation simply does not facilitate power-sharing. So there likely remains a dominance of professional power, and the inclusion of peer helping merely augments the system rather than modifies its locus of power that remains within some hierarchy among human service professionals.

Peer helpers, like peer support specialists, may simply hold an ambiguous status within such a culture. The system itself may overlook the identity transformation taking place among people who serve as peer support specialists, and limit their career paths. The system may also overlook how the formalization of peer support roles may alter profoundly the relationships among the incumbents of those roles and their peers. In other words, peers may see those incumbents through an altered lens that confuses how they should relate to those individuals. Do they relate to them as trusted peers, or as quasi-professionals who may be seeking to expand professional control or system control over their lives?

Extension can occur when new support systems, not under the direct control of consumers, require their substantial involvement in the operation of that particular support system. Organizationally, the system extends into domains that the established human service model itself cannot readily address because of resource constraints or the diminished status such helping may hold within the social or human service hierarchy (Moxley, 2002). Consistent with the moral treatment of late nineteenth and early twentieth-century mental hygiene, these systems may literally extend into domains that human problems, like mental illness, are seen to weaken, at least from the perspective of human service professionals. Thus, extending into housing, work, and the organization of daily life may serve as a way of socializing otherwise deviant people into normative roles.

Wiseman's work suggests such an outcome of extension through the creation of specialized environments that either remove people from the mainstream or erect barriers, particularly physical ones, separating certain groups from the mainstream. The models themselves may devolve into dehumanization in which participants are limited in the opportunities they have available to them. Alternatively, the model may help people regain their confidence, gain skills they want to achieve, pursue the aims they wish for themselves, or experience protection from what too often can be a cruel world.

A progressive policy likely comes about under conditions of reform. There is a perception by community members, human service professionals, families of recipients, and recipients themselves that something is not right, or even seriously wrong. People may experience harm at the proverbial hands of the system. There may be media exposes concerning the troubles of the system. Deaths may have occurred. Advocates may prevail in court when they are victorious in pressing the system to change.

The system may change as a result of coercive forces, and progressive strategies emerge, ones based in humanism seeking to offer recipients, particularly those who have experienced the original neglect first-hand, are offered new options for social support, opportunities, and personal development. Some systems may move from crisis to reform in cycles. Progressive practice may devolve into system decline, only to reemerge as "old wine in a new bottle," through processes of the rejuvenation, or renaissance of the system.

Some systems may possess a different approach to development. They may purposively embrace new practices and encode them into their cultures of care, treatment, and support. Those systems do not wait for crisis as a coercive stimulus orchestrating introspection and subsequent change. They alter themselves by design and to do so they prospect for potentially new approaches to the care they offer recipients. In this sense, the system may not radically alter how it operates, but through incremental change, realized largely through the adoption of what they see as promising practices, system representatives select building blocks to alter the relationships between professionals and recipients. The resulting incremental change here is in a sense a kind of system reform.

Progressive reform, therefore, operates within the system. It legitimizes the system as it is altering membership qualities of recipients and professionals, adding new statuses and roles for recipients, and creating environments operated by recipients themselves, involving options like recipient-controlled drop-in centers, employment options, clubs, and socialization opportunities.

Radical Policy Strategies

Alternatively, radical strategies may involve a shifting of power into a network of peers who follow natural group processes in the evolution of the culture and politics of alternative support entities emanating out of two potential policy strategies: *enhancement* and *substitution*. I organize both strategies within a radical value set because they offer a critical engagement of existing human service and societal arrangements, incorporate a counter-narrative guiding action, and seek to empower the person as a social actor.

Radical strategies make sense in the light of human management models that are controlling human beings, limiting their freedom, enforcing negative stereotypes, and reducing options for human development. Wiseman captures such a human management model in *Public Housing*, and especially in *Titicut Follies*. The greater society sets the framework of worthiness and merit, and allocates options to people based on its privileged status. That status enables the system to degrade the lives of those who possess certain social attachments, like race, who are seen as a threat to the society, or who are seen merely as surplus and, as a result, the greater society has determined them to be unneeded and unwanted.

Radical strategies bring legitimacy of the system into question, incorporate critiques of existing arrangements, and frame human services as a social institution expressing a dark side of the greater society. The questioning brings into focus how too often human professionals serve social control purposes, and what previously I call progressive responses are from a radical perspective merely a smoke-screen set up by a society that legitimizes considerable neglect and abuse.

Enhancement can operate through an enabling culture in which the status of the participant shifts from one of recipient to an empowered actor whose aim is to bring about a resolution they want for themselves. The agent gains control over the framing and selection of issues and the specification of desired outcomes (Freddolino et al., 2004; Moxley & Hyduk, 2003). The enhancement of status here is a key aspect of radical practice. The strategy empowers both the status of the person as decision-maker and their role within a culture that views issues as products of social forces like deprivation, discrimination, oppression, and marginalization (Moxley & Washington, 2009). Enhancement as a strategy implicates social forces and focuses on those institutions, organizations, and actors who bring about damage as a result of those social forces and the arrangements they bring about, such as mass incarceration.

Substitution replaces existing human service arrangements for those participants who affiliate with such alternative options. Diverse options can foster new conceptions of the participants' identities perhaps helping them see themselves as objects of abuse and neglect inherent in a violation of their basic human rights. Such identity formation can embrace other experiences emanating from class, ethnicity, gender, race, age, and sexual orientation. The narratives can reveal how important it is to understand how social structural factors intersect to create vulnerability (Washington & Moxley, 2009). Still, substitution as a policy strategy may foster new resources mediated by alternative outsider organizations, and novel pathways can emerge for participants who can realize quality of life outcomes involving income, housing, food, education, affiliation, personal and cultural development, and well-being.

Those embodying radical ideas and constructs may look for avenues to assist survivors shape such entities. Human service professionals who come to embrace such strategies will likely witness their own transformation. They may come to see themselves as external advocates who represent the wishes of the people they assist. They may locate themselves on the margins or periphery of a particular system practicing rights protection and advocacy, occupying roles in public interest law firms, or participating in support systems unrecognized or delegitimized by those centers of power representing commonly accepted ideas about human vulnerability, and the desirable or acceptable response to such vulnerability. Practitioners and organizations embodying radical strategies may push at established human service systems to reform if not revolutionize their institutional cultures.

Using models and practices from community organization, the radical practitioner can collaborate with other participants in the co-creation of social enclaves that stand as mutual support and self-help entities within a community as alternatives to established human service systems. Those enclaves can incubate alternative or counter narratives about the plight of those who experience what is for them a socially manufactured degradation.

Veterans organized outside of a military base may incubate this narrative on a daily basis, growing a perspective that is not conciliatory but demanding. Orchestrating those demands may occur through public awareness campaigns or protests launched against the entities the enclave members see as responsible for the creation and exacerbation of their plight. Often the intent of radical strategies is to bring into public consciousness the realities of public neglect and even abuse. While the media may create the expose motivating progressive institutional reform, radical strategists likely see themselves as the authors of such exposes. They can use the media as their own vehicle for exposing what is wrong for them and what they find unacceptable.

Animating the radical strategies are two concepts about social status. One is my use of the concept of *degraded status*. I invoke this concept to amplify the idea that social welfare policy can (intentionally or unintentionally) create situations of daily life that are themselves degraded but that the society justifies by the qualities of those individuals. Officials can rationalize this degradation as "just desserts" for the failure of some people to practice those values and virtues the society endorses. Agents of the greater society may invoke disease, illness, or impairment as a violation of purity. This absence of purity may invoke dread within the greater society further justifying the removal and isolation of an unwanted group. However, as Douglas (1966) observes in her book, *Purity and Danger*, a society's enforcement of standards of purity must address their violation. Human services may be the way in which society addresses impurity, or the violation of those standards that define normality.

Mainstream actors may experience an aesthetic violation—the sheer sight of deviant individuals could assault the senses (and sensibilities) of those actors. The intentional or even unintentional deprivation enforced by social welfare policy and its agents can further create the degradation experienced by those labeled deviant, further setting in motion a violation of the senses and sensibilities of mainstream actors.

A second concept I invoke involves *diminished status*. As society strips away those resources people require to survive and to enjoy their lives, as it justifies deprivation, and rationalizes mistreatment, diminished status occurs because people do not have the standing before social institutions to demand adequate and just treatment. Weakening their status is the absence of human rights, particularly what Eleanor Roosevelt came to call social rights (Glendon, 2001). Eleanor pushed her husband to recognize those rights as a bill of social rights, the absence of which is so apparent in the Constitution of the United States. Those rights would recognize what Thomas Jefferson saw as a modicum of prosperity all human beings should come to enjoy. But Eleanor's vision did not prevail. Many people, particularly in the United States, do not have automatic claims as a function of their citizenship to life necessities like housing, income, health care, food, and housing.

Radical policies would articulate, legitimize, or promote such claims. They would recognize the standing of all people to make claims on social institutions for what Jefferson came to call a modicum of prosperity. Ultimately, given the centrality of those claims to human health and prosperity, radical strategists and practitioners would come to advance social status to heighten the claims people can make on the greater society. These claims would manifest themselves in the empowerment of status so that the social rights of people would not be diminished. For radical practitioners the strategies of enhancement and substitution would empower people by advancing their standing and claims for social goods or benefits before social institutions.

Conclusion: Consumerism and Social Change of Human Services

Consumerism and its manifestation in the lives of consumer recipient and survivor can influence how social change can occur in human services. Consumerism in established systems reveals how reform can occur when those systems build alternatives for consumers within their institutional and operational cultures. For consumers, role options previously unavailable to them can raise their expectations about how they could actuate helping roles as peers. They can bring to those systems a form of expertise oftentimes unavailable to professionals whose knowledge may objectify recipients in the process of care.

Armed with personal experience and with a knowledge base that is difficult to gain through professional education, consumer recipients can be well positioned to bring forms of understanding that can enrich those systems, and expand their spheres of competence. As I have pointed out previously, however, there are some potential pitfalls for consumers whose roles transform through the addition of responsibilities for the provision of social support to their peers. Surmounting these pitfalls, and amplifying the contributions consumer recipients can make, holds the promise of humanizing a system, and can counter dehumanization.

By creating novel consumer roles, creating peer operated support systems, offering alternative interactional routines among recipients, and between recipients and professionals, and deepening the options available to recipients, a human service system can realize some appreciable internal change. Consumerism can be linked to a grander internal system change program resulting in the alteration of organizational culture.

Strident and adversarial survivors can serve as a reminder that collective responses to human need are limited in most societies. The existence of prejudice, discrimination, and degraded environments are part and parcel of diminished status. The abridgment of voice can escalate frustration and anger for people seeking a better life unfettered by inadequate resources, inappropriate and unnecessary labeling, harassment at the hands of officials, and closed and/or nonexistent opportunity structures.

Survivors themselves can model new ways of meeting human needs, and reveal deprivation and mistreatment. Street theater, performance, protest, and confrontation may remind social control officials, like police, that they are arresting and detaining people whose bodies, minds, and emotions may be different from what the mainstream prefers. Those officials may come to think that they are compensating for poor social policy in which people's needs go unrecognized or their voices go unheard. Perhaps the last thing police officers want to do is to arrest people who are exercising their voice in contexts in which policymakers will not listen.

Activism is now a common form of practice, especially in societies coming to grips with an activist citizenry, and a strong if not bold civil society. Deep respect for this form of self-expression, particularly at group levels, has been institutionalized in what George Soros calls open societies, and is gaining ground in closed societies. Survivors can remind policymakers and those who are enfranchised with the responsibilities for the management of human groups that human decency involving respect for the perspectives of outsiders, the importance of dignity, and the adequacy of provision is central to creating an inclusive society. Consumerism and social inclusion are intimately connected.

References

Douglas, M. (1966). *Purity and danger*. Routledge.

Freddolino, P., Moxley, D., & Hyduk, C. (2004). A differential model of advocacy in social work practice. *Families in Society, 85*(1), 119–128.

Glendon, M. A. (2001). *A world made new: Eleanor Roosevelt and the universal declaration of human rights*. Random House.

Grant, B. K. (2006). *Five films by Frederick Wiseman*. University of California Press.

Moxley, D. (2002, October). The emergence and attributes of second-generation community support services for persons with serious mental illness: Implications for case management. *Journal of Social Work in Disability and Rehabilitation, 1*(2), 25–52.

Moxley, D., & Hyduk, C. (2003, January). The logic of personal advocacy with older adults and its implications for program management in community gerontology. *Administration in Social Work, 27*(4), 5–23.

Moxley, D., & Washington, O. (2009). The role of advocacy assessment and action in resolving health compromising stress in the lives of older African American homeless women. In L. Napier & P. Waters (Eds.), *Social work and global health inequalities: Policy and practice developments*. Policy Press.

Washington, O., & Moxley, D. (2009). "I Have Three Strikes against Me": Narratives of plight and efficacy among older African American homeless women and their implications for engaged inquiry. In S. Evans (Ed.), *African Americans and community engagement in higher education*. State University of New York Press.

Wiseman, F. (1967). *Titicut Follies*. Zipporah Films.

Wiseman, F. (1968). *High School I*. Zipporah Films.

Wiseman, F. (1975). *Welfare*. Zipporah Films.

Wiseman, F. (1986). *Adjustment and Work*. Zipporah Films.

Wiseman, F. (1994). *High School II*. Zipporah Films.

Wiseman, F. (1997). *Public Housing*. Zipporah Films.

8

Consumerism as an Enduring Social Force in Human Services

Introduction

What is in store for consumerism in the near future, as social welfare policy in both the developing and developed worlds grapple with aging, poverty, and long-term illness or disability, all within the context of climate change shaping human need and its fulfillment? Confining health promotion both within the developed and developing worlds to the mitigation of disease and illness, or even its prevention, cannot be the sole solution in advancing the well-being of whole populations. In the developing world, the promise of social development links social policy advancement in covering various populations, or whole communities, to address their well-being through local options for advancing the immediate issues that communities and neighborhoods as well as other human settlements face on a daily basis (Simeon et al., 2019).

This linkage is a promising one fostering civic engagement, participation, and organizational development at lower levels within a given society. The emergence of local organizations within urban, rural, and frontier contexts founded by citizens themselves reflects one of the driving forces in consumerism: the involvement of common people in finding solutions

© The Author(s), under exclusive license to Springer Nature Singapore Pte Ltd. 2021   **115**
D. P. Moxley, *Consumerism in the Human Services*,
https://doi.org/10.1007/978-981-16-7192-0_8

for advancing the quality of environment and quality of life in their daily interactions within group life. Here group life may be one of the most important aspects of advancing well-being. Operating in small groups especially within democratic structures, people can thrive not only through their face-to-face (or cybernetic) exchanges with others, but also by taking joint action to improve collective well-being in local situations.

This joint action is the basis of consumerism in the greater society. That people would choose to align themselves to address inequities, especially through amplifying their perspectives (revealing the importance of voice in transactions occurring between individuals and greater societal structures) reinforces consumerism within societies. The multiplication of the voice of individuals, and its coalescence into movements, are certainly a force for change in society. Some critics may only consider these movements as indicative of identity politics. But locality-based organizing and the social innovation it can produce is an important product of such efforts. Groups may continue to advance their identities, but local communities may themselves offer integration across groups offering coherence and harmony within localities.

The founding of social development organizations at local levels are expressions of a grander idea behind civil society: that there is another sector of society other than business and government that has a strong interest in addressing human well-being. Social development organizations are now well rooted in the African and South Asia experience, are broader in scope than specialized nonprofit or nongovernmental organizations, and are focused on locality development. Locality development implicates the development of local leadership, broad-based institutional, group, and individual involvement, and a focus on local issues that are likely reflective of greater social issues visible on national levels. In this sense, locality development is glocal. It can recognize that global issues operate at local levels, and that local solutions may have global implications.

Consumerism as Activism

What does this mean for consumerism? Underlying consumerism is the idea of activism. Activists serve a sentinel function—they likely anticipate what the broader society will finally recognize as an issue. Activists therefore produce information for the greater society and correct for institutional denial or obfuscation of reality or truth. Activists are one of the greatest resources for social change. Consumerism incorporates social activism, and can support people whose voice is tamped down by greater societal actors or structures. As I have noted in previous chapters of this monograph, consumerism is about voice and dissent. It is about participation within particular social systems, like human services, or it is about dissent, perhaps catalyzing action against that system resulting in the development of novel institutions. Such alternatives can prefigure what is now occurring and become what is common in the future. Activism and innovation may be inextricably linked. Through such linkages society can experience a press for social change even though there is a lag in how the greater society responds in immediate situations.

By alternative I am referring to group life or organizations that operate by values and routines that may contrast sharply with existing societal arrangements. Some may say those arrangements are deviant since they do not fall in line with an existing paradigm, like viewing mental illness exclusively through a medical lens. There is a good case for approaching mental illness using a medical model. But even with this kind of orientation, mental illness produces numerous social and cultural consequences necessitating a broader approach to offering social support. This broader approach may incorporate a concept of health that differs from the narrower idea used within many societies.

The adoption of this broader approach, a broader lens, is at the root of consumerism. Consumerism may correct for narrow perspectives adopted by societal decision-makers who especially want to control public expenditures. Consumerism pursues accountability (visible in the lawsuits of a previous era revealing societal abuse or neglect) and social innovation broadens social roles (and power or influence) within established human service systems and their composite organizations.

Consumerism as Social and Organizational Innovation

Consumerism within human services is here to stay and will continue to evolve in its levels and forms of social innovation. Five forms of innovation are salient as one examines consumerism.

- It broadens both professional and societal recognition of the importance of mutual support among people experiencing certain conditions. Mutual support has broadened an understanding of healing factors operating in illness, and it has broadened insight into the problematic and health-threatening dynamics of isolation as a result of societal stigma.
- It reveals the limitations of professionalism. As human and health service professionals became concerned with efficiency of care and volume as well as the business aspects of care, consumerism built alternative options for people, especially in four ways: the importance of social support, the creation of new explanations of factors exacerbating human problems, the production of new information sources, and the creation of new accountabilities for human and health professionals. Here the consumerist critique—that professionals could never offer a framework for fully addressing or offering the solutions to the issues people experience—challenges what professionals can offer. And, unbridled professionalism can create negative consequences even as professionals sought to do good by the people they assist.
- It reduces the sanctity of professional power, and moderates the exercise of this power within contexts of care or even within society as a whole. Consumerism established a sense of professional responsibility for responding quickly to those who experience serious illness and disability. A good example here is the consumer movement in AIDS as the movement itself pressured the National Institutes of Health to change its protocol for addressing the AIDS crisis. The innovation here was an augmentation of advocacy in a social problem space in which people suffering with AIDS (both its medical realities and social consequences) began a countermovement to a grander societal narra-

tive in which people with AIDS were seen as the problem and the danger.

- It also broadens the roles and hopefully the opportunity structures available to people coping with various issues, including physical, cognitive, emotional, or behavioral ones. Such role change implicates how professionals and consumers, as well as policymakers, come to see expertise. From the perspective of a negative stance or critique, the development of new roles recognizes the limitations of professionals and traditional structures that can organize rigid responses to recipients. That rigidity can reduce access and appropriateness of care, and it can obviate engagement and relationship building between recipients and health professionals. And that rigidity can instill distrust in recipients. On a positive side, the alliance between professionals and people serving in peer support roles, or those who may see themselves as prosumers (those who hold dual roles involving professional role and consumer role) can correct for the negative aspects of professionalism and instill practices indicative of a consumer-centered culture of care or support, Thus, as what my colleague Dr. Carol Mowbray and I referred to as "consumers as providers" can strengthen outreach, particularly working at the street level, engagement of people in their households, and on the streets, and the creation of support systems in which people's values and aims are central to the provision of support and care from professionals.

- And, it broadens the rights of consumers over their access to care, over their say in their treatment, over their right to adequate and necessary information about the care they are receiving, and about their options to criticize their treatment. These rights also reflect an expansion of the role of the recipient in care or treatment settings. This augmentation of rights has lessened the use of the term of patient or even client in human service organizations. The range of ways some organizations refer to people who receive care is quite broad. They may be called patients, consumers, recipients, users, or clients. Each has its own strengths and limitations, but what the range indicates is that consumerism has introduced considerable ambiguity into human services. This ambiguity may be a transition state in which consumers in human and health services may finally gain some semblance of control over the resources they receive and over the conduct and accountability of professionals. The emergence of consumer control suggests that the discretion of professionals will be increasingly narrowed. Not only can people enjoy this control over their decision-making, but the information base supporting this control is expansive. Consumers can bring into transactions with professionals considerable information, insight, and understanding.

Critique of Professional Privilege

The survivor movement has intensified the critique of professional privilege. Certainly, survivors have amplified the critique of professionals and society, particularly in societal abuse or neglect. A grand narrative of the survivor movement is the assertion of its members that professionals are complicit in the social control agenda of the greater society. This social control manifests itself in a number of ways involving: (1) the behavioral control of people with certain qualities through oversight such as enhanced case management within human service systems, (2) the geographic isolation of people in what could be considered ghettoes reinforced by limited entitlements pushing people into poverty or living at a survival level, (3) stigmatization and compounded stigmatization thereby expanding the social distance between people, (4) rights deprivation and confinement evident in the incarceration of people with certain labels, (5) the exclusion of people from opportunity structures so they can escape the deprivation they face, and (6) the degradation of environments.

Still, consumer recipients may recognize the limitations of professionalism when they assert the unique perspectives they bring to the provision of care. That perspective can encompass a direct experience with issues recipients bring to human services when they are searching for assistance. Reception by an experienced recipient, one who knows how the organization really functions, may help newcomers to make better decisions, and get the care they want. An experienced recipient who knows how the organization works and can help people travel a course of action productively is consistent with the navigator movement in human services. Navigators' expertise crystallizes from their experience and their direct engagement of human issues at a personal level. For newcomers, however, navigators may simply introduce more ambiguity into the care process—do navigators take the side of the recipient or does their presence indicate the limitations of the human service system: that it is very complex and the function of the navigator is to ensure that someone does not get lost, give up, or get entangled in processes that are counterproductive for someone searching for assistance.

Artificial Intelligence (AI) may temper professionalism considerably (Susskind & Susskind, 2015). Consumers will increasingly possess more knowledge about issues they face, and the organizations that address these issues. Consumers may come into organizations with considerable information about what they need, and the available responses they require to resolve or remedy the issues they face. Consumerism is tied to information, and there are ample systems of information that equip consumers with the information they require to achieve ends they value. AI will likely redefine professions, especially in the human services, and will make some professions redundant as organizations install information and decision systems that substitute for professional judgment. Given the enduring information revolution the globe is experiencing, AI may be a new layer of capacity that empowers human service consumers, individually and collectively.

Conclusion: The Conditions That Drive Consumerism

What are the conditions under which consumerism emerges and gains ground? Perhaps one of the most influential forces is bureaucracies that become unresponsive to the people to whom they should be responsive. Bureaucratic reform emanating out of consumer pressure to become more responsive can drive consumerism. Inherent in at least a person-centered approach, those bureaucracies not only take into consideration and take seriously what people need (or actually want for themselves but they take the social attachments of the people they serve seriously as well. This means ethnicity, race, regional, and historic concerns become important for those bureaucracies). And other social attachments factor into the equation of responsiveness—like language, socio-economic status, and cultural identities. Why do these matter? Because it is those kinds of attachments that foster identity.

Understanding that identity is critical for responsiveness of a bureaucracy to the people it assists. When responsiveness is nonexistent or breaks down, conflict can evolve between those with the sanction to help and those who are in need. When the organization neglects those individuals in need then problems escalate. When the organization outright abuses people then this is a more sinister matter. Responsiveness and consumerism align, an intersection especially important when the social welfare apparatus within a society is mediated by bureaucracies.

Related here is institutional breakdown. In the case of such breakdown, major social institutions and their representatives become neglectful of the people they are sanctioned to help. In the United States, the situation of veterans is instructive here. What is experienced or even perceived as an unresponsive Veterans Administration may signal an uncaring society, one in which veterans are seen as unimportant or are even dismissed as people who can make claims based on their service. Institutional neglect may sever the contract between people who feel they are deserving and those who allocate rights, benefits, and opportunities. That the issue with military veterans still lingers in the United States suggests that American society has not really empowered the status of the veteran, their partners, and their families. In the case of combat exposed veterans, the violation of this contract fuels consumerism in some interesting ways.

Consistent with the theory and framework I offer in this monograph, there is a conciliatory approach in which government-sponsored veterans' programs hire more veterans, place them in responsible roles, blend professional and peer support, and expand support veterans can receive, like enhanced social services and advocacy for those veterans who experience homelessness. In addition, there is evidence for a confrontational approach in which veterans protest their mistreatment linked to neglect. It is this narrative that forms under conditions of dissent. And, finally there is evidence of withdrawal. Here veterans form their own mutual support organizations and address the expanded needs of the people whom they care for and about. Veterans help veterans and see their withdrawal as a form of rejection of the prevailing arrangements of governmental funded social, health, and rehabilitation services.

This example underscores the diversity of consumerism and its various vectors. Each offers a particular culture of human engagement in relationship to government and those arrangements government puts in place to address human need. I underscore the idea of arrangements since influencing those are archetypes of how a society sees people in need and the paradigms, they find acceptable in addressing those needs. Archetypes may frame those who have certain needs in pejorative ways and, as a result, offer particular paradigms for managing that need. The deeply seeded perspectives of society regarding human need and the paradigms those perspectives produce offer the ultimate rationale for consumerism.

References

Simeon, A., Butterfield, A. K., & Moxley, D. P. (2019). Locality-based social development: A theoretical perspective for social work. In M. Payne & E. R. Hall (Eds.), *Routledge Handbook of social work theory* (pp. 294–307). Routledge.

Susskind, R., & Susskind, D. (2015). *The future of the professions: How technology will transform the work of human experts*. New York.

References

Allen, F. A. (1981). *The decline of the rehabilitative ideal: Penal policy and social purpose*. Yale University Press.

Anthony, W. A. (1993). Recovery from mental illness: The guiding vision of the mental health service system in the 1990s. *Psychosocial Rehabilitation Journal, 16*, 11–23.

Anthony, W. A. (2004). The principle of personhood: The field's transcendent principle. *Psychiatric Rehabilitation Journal, 27*, 205.

Basaglia, F. (1982). Institutions of violence. In N. Scheper-Hughes & A. M. Lovell (Eds.), *Psychiatry inside-out: Selected writings of Franco Basaglia* (pp. 58–85). Columbia University Press.

Beers, C. (1908). *A mind that found itself: An autobiography*. Longman.

Bockhoven, J. S. (1956). Moral treatment in American psychiatry. *Journal of Nervous and Mental Disease, 124*, 292–321.

Borg, M., & Davidson, L. (2007). The nature of recovery as lived in everyday experience. *Journal of Mental Health, 16*, 1–12.

Brown, T. J. (1998). *Dorothea Dix: New England reformer*. Harvard University Press.

Caplan, G. (1964). *Principles of preventive psychiatry*. Basic Books.

Caplan, G. (1974). *Support systems and community mental health.* Behavioral Publications.

Chamberlain, J. (1990). The ex-patients' movement: Where we've been and where we're going. *Journal of Mind and Behavior, 11,* 323–336.

Charlton, J. (2000). *Nothing about us without us: Disability oppression and empowerment.* University of California Press.

Corrigan, P. W., Mueser, K. T., Bond, G. R., Drake, R. E., & Solomon, P. (2008). *Principles and practice of psychiatric rehabilitation: An empirical approach.* Guilford.

Dain, N. (1980). *Clifford W. Beers: Advocate for the Insane.* University of Pittsburgh Press.

Davidson, L., Kirk, T., Rockholz, P., et al. (2007). Creating a recovery-oriented system of behavioral health care: Moving from concept to reality. *Psychiatric Rehabilitation Journal, 31,* 23–31.

Davidson, L., Rakfeldt, J., & Strauss, J. (2010). *The roots of the recovery movement.* Wiley.

Davidson, L., & White, W. (2007). The concept of recovery as an organizing principle for integrating mental health and addiction services. *Journal of Behavioral Health Services and Research, 34,* 109–120.

Douglas, M. (1966). *Purity and danger.* Routledge.

Douglas, M. (1982). *Risk and culture.* University of California Press.

Douglas, M. (1986). *How institutions think.* Syracuse University Press.

Douglas, M., & Ney, S. (1998). *Missing person: A critique of personhood in the social sciences.* Russel Sage Foundation.

Eco, U. (2007). *On ugliness.* Rizzoli.

Feen-Calligan, H., Washington, O., & Moxley, D. P. (2009). Homelessness among older African American women: Interpreting a serious social issue through the arts in community based participatory action research. *New Solutions: Journal of Environmental and Occupational Health Policy, 19*(4), 423–448.

Felice, W. (1996). *Taking suffering seriously: The importance of collective human rights.* SUNY Press.

Freddolino, P., Moxley, D., & Hyduk, C. (2004). A differential model of advocacy in social work practice. *Families in Society, 85*(1), 119–128.

Glendon, M. A. (2001). *A world made new: Eleanor Roosevelt and the universal declaration of human rights.* Random House.

Glickman, M., & Flannery, M. (1996). *Fountain house: Portraits of lives reclaimed from mental illness.* Hazelden.

Grant, B. K. (2006). *Five films by Frederick Wiseman.* University of California Press.

Hirschman, A. O. (1970). *Exit, voice, and loyalty: Responses to decline in firms, organizations and states.* Harvard University Press.

Jackson, R. L. (2000). *The clubhouse model: Empowering applications of theory to generalist practice.* Brooks Cole.

Johnson, A. B. (1990). *Out of Bedlam: The truth about deinstitutionalization.* Basic Books.

Joint Commission on Mental Illness and Health. (1961). *Action for mental health.* Basic Books.

Jones, C. (2000). *The making of an activist: Stitching a revolution.* Harper.

Kateb, G. (2011). *Human dignity.* Belknap Harvard.

Mowbray, C., Moxley, D., & Collins, M. E. (1998, November). Consumers as mental health providers: First person accounts of benefits and limitations. *The Journal of Behavioral Health Services and Research, 25*(4), 397–411.

Mowbray, C., Moxley, D., Jasper, C., & Howell, L. (Eds.). (1997). *Consumers as providers in psychiatric rehabilitation.* IAPSRS.

Mowbray, C., Moxley, D., & Van Tosh, L. (2001, May). Changing roles for primary consumers in community psychiatry. In J. Talbot & R. Hales (Eds.), *Textbook of administrative psychiatry: New concepts for a changing behavioral health system* (2nd ed.). American Psychiatric Publishing, Inc..

Mowbray, C., Strauch-Brown, K., Furlong-Norman, K., & Sullivan Soydan, A. (2002). *Supported education & psychiatric rehabilitation: Models and methods.* USPRA.

Mowbray, C. T., & Moxley, D. P. (1997a). Futures for empowerment of consumer role innovation. In C. T. Mowbray, D. Moxley, C. Jasper, & L. Davis (Eds.), *Consumers as providers in psychiatric rehabilitation.* International Association of Psychosocial Rehabilitation Services.

Mowbray, C. T., & Moxley, D. P. (1997b). A framework for organizing consumers as providers in psychiatric rehabilitation. In C. T. Mowbray, D. Moxley, C. Jasper, & L. Davis (Eds.), *Consumers as providers in psychiatric rehabilitation.* International Association of Psychosocial Rehabilitation Services.

Mowbray, C. T., & Moxley, D. P. (1997c). Consumers as providers: Themes and success factors. In C. T. Mowbray, D. Moxley, C. Jasper, & L. Davis (Eds.), *Consumers as providers in psychiatric rehabilitation.* International Association of Psychosocial Rehabilitation Services Press.

Moxley, D. (2002, October). The emergence and attributes of second-generation community support services for persons with serious mental illness: Implications for case management. *Journal of Social Work in Disability and Rehabilitation, 1*(2), 25–52.

Moxley, D., & Freddolino, P. (1990, September). A model of advocacy for promoting client self-determination in psychosocial rehabilitation. *Psychosocial Rehabilitation Journal, 14*(2), 69–82.

Moxley, D., & Freddolino, P. (1994, June). Client-driven advocacy and psychiatric disability: A Model for social work practice. *Journal of Sociology and Social Welfare, 21*(2), 98–108.

Moxley, D., & Hyduk, C. (2003, January). The logic of personal advocacy with older adults and its implications for program management in community gerontology. *Administration in Social Work, 27*(4), 5–23.

Moxley, D., & Paul, M. (2005, May). Advocacy and guardianship. In W. Crimando & T. F. Riggar (Eds.), *Community resources: A practical guide for human service professionals* (pp. 200–217). Waveland Press.

Moxley, D., & Washington, O. (2009). The role of advocacy assessment and action in resolving health compromising stress in the lives of older African American homeless women. In L. Napier & P. Waters (Eds.), *Social work and global health inequalities: Policy and practice developments*. Policy Press.

Moxley, D. P., Feen-Calligan, H., & Washington, O. G. M. (2012, July). Lessons learned from three projects linking social work, the arts and humanities. *Social Work Education: the International Journal, 31*(6), 703–723.

Moxley, D. P., & Mowbray, C. T. (1997, April). Consumers as providers: Social forces and factors legitimizing role innovation in psychiatric rehabilitation. In C. T. Mowbray, D. Moxley, C. Jasper, & L. Davis (Eds.), *Consumers as providers in psychiatric rehabilitation*. International Association of Psychosocial Rehabilitation Services.

Nader, R. (1967). Keynote address presented to the consumer assembly. In R. Nader (Ed.), *The ralph Nader reader*. Seven Stories Press.

Nader, R. (2012). Unsafe at any speed. In E. Bruun & J. Crosby (Eds.), *The American experience: The history and culture of the United States*. Black Dog & Leventhal Press.

Nader, R., Green, M., & Seligman, J. (1976). Who rules the giant corporation? *Business and Society Review*, Summer.

O'Brien, J. (2002). Person-centered planning as a contributing factor in organizational and social change. *Research and Practice in Persistent and Severe Disability, 27*, 261–264.

Pitzer, A. (2017). *One long night: A global history of concentration campus*. Little, Brown.

Rieff, D. (2002). *A bed for the night: Humanitarianism in crisis*. Simon & Schuster.

Roosevelt, T. (2012). The national should assume power of regulation over all corporations. In E. Bruun & J. Crosby (Eds.), *The American experience: The history and culture of the United States*. Black Dog & Leventhal Press.

Rosen, M. (2012). *Dignity: Its history and meaning*. Harvard University Press.

Ryan, W. (1976). *Blaming the victim* (Revised and updated edition). Vintage.

Schein, E. (with Peter Schein) (2016). *Organizational leadership and culture* (5th ed.). Wiley.

Scheper-Hughes, N., & Lovell, A. M. (1986). Breaking the circuit of social control: Lessons in public psychiatry from Italy and Franco Basaglia. *Social Science and Medicine, 23*, 159–178.

Shotwell, A. (2016). *Against purity: Living ethically in compromised times*. University of Minnesota Press.

Simeon, A., Butterfield, A. K., & Moxley, D. P. (2019). Locality-based social development: A theoretical perspective for social work. In M. Payne & E. R. Hall (Eds.), *Routledge Handbook of social work theory* (pp. 294–307). Routledge.

Stein, L., & Test, M. (1980). *Alternative to mental hospital treatment*. Plenum.

Stern, G. (2012). School superintendents call for tougher gun control, mental health funding. *Lohud.com*. Retrieved December 20, 2012, from http://www.lohud.com/article/20121231/NEWS/312310066/School-superintendents-call-tougher-gun-control-mental-health-funding

Susskind, R., & Susskind, D. (2015). *The future of the professions: How technology will transform the work of human experts*. New York.

Swarbrick, M., & Schmidt, L. (Eds.). (2010). *People in recovery as providers of psychiatric rehabilitation*. USPRA.

Teplin, L., McClelland, G., Abram, K., & Weiner, D. (2005). Crime victimization in adults with severe mental illness: Comparison with the National Crime Victimization Survey. *Archives of General Psychiatry, 62*, 911–921.

Turner, J. C., & TenHoor, W. J. (1978). The NIMH community support program: Pilot approach to a needed social reform. *Schizophrenia Bulletin, 4*, 319–348.

United States Department of Health and Human Services. (1999). *Mental health: A report of the Surgeon General*. Author.

United States Department of Health and Human Services. (2003). *Achieving the promise: Transforming mental health care in America, President's New Freedom Commission on Mental Health*. Final Report. USDHHS.

United States Department of Health and Human Services. (2005). *Transforming mental health care in America, Federal action agenda: First steps*. Author.

Viebeck, E. (2012, December 21). Catholic bishops call for gun control, mental health reforms. *Healthwatch*. Retrieved December 24, 2012, from http://the-hill.com/blogs/healthwatch/mental-health/274235-catholic-bishops-call-for-gun-control-mental-health-reform

Waldron, J. (2015). *Dignity, rank, and rights*. New York.

Washington, O., & Moxley, D. (2008). Telling my story: From narrative to exhibit in illuminating the lived experience of homelessness among older African American women. *Journal of Health Psychology, 13*(2), 154–165.

Washington, O., & Moxley, D. (2009). "I Have Three Strikes against Me": Narratives of plight and efficacy among older African American homeless women and their implications for engaged inquiry. In S. Evans (Ed.), *African Americans and community engagement in higher education*. State University of New York Press.

Weisberg, S. E. (2009). *Barney Frank*. University of Massachusetts Press.

Wiseman, F. (1967). *Titicut Follies*. Zipporah Films.

Wiseman, F. (1968). *High School I*. Zipporah Films.

Wiseman, F. (1975). *Welfare*. Zipporah Films.

Wiseman, F. (1986). *Adjustment and Work*. Zipporah Films.

Wiseman, F. (1994). *High School II*. Zipporah Films.

Wiseman, F. (1997). *Public Housing*. Zipporah Films.

Yarbrough, T. (1981). *Judge Frank Johnson and human rights in Alabama*. University of Alabama Press.

Index

Printed in the United States
by Baker & Taylor Publisher Services